...and another thing

Rants, raves, and information you can use on everything from drug company greed to Vitamin C

A collection of the all time best HSI e-Alerts

from the desk of Jenny Thompson.

Jenny Thompson
with John Averill

...and another thing:
A collection of the all time best HSI e-Alerts

Published by Agora Health Books

Alice Wessendorf, Managing editor
Gerrit Wessendorf, Cover and book design

ISBN 1-891434-29-2

Printed in the United States of America

Agora Health Books
819 N. Charles Street
Baltimore, Maryland 21201
www.agorahealthbooks.com

...and another thing:
A collection of the all time best HSI e-Alerts

Jenny Thompson
with
John Averill

Agora Health Books
Baltimore, Maryland

DISCLAIMER

All material in this publication is provided for information only and may not be construed as medical advice or instruction. The information and opinions provided in this book are believed to be accurate and sound, based on the best judgment available to the authors, but readers who fail to consult with appropriate health authorities assume the risk of any injuries. No action should be taken based solely on the contents of this publication; instead, readers should consult appropriate health professionals on any matter relating to their health and well-being. The publisher is not responsible for errors or omissions.

Table of Contents

Dedication

Every day, I get a good number of e-mails complimenting the e-Alert and commending me for writing it. Every day, I forward those e-mails to the team around me that really makes it happen. So, a big thank you...to John Averill, Scott Schoberg, Barb Ogden and Corin Mauldin. Without them, the e-Alert would just be an e- and you might not get it at all.

Yes, those are the people that make the e-Alert happen every day. But the reason the e-Alert happens is not because of me, or John, or Scott. It's because of:

Kate and Carmen T.
George L.
Bonnie Z.
Chuck
Eleanor L.
Richard Z.
Andy B.
Tom B.
Flip B. (did we really need the last initial, you might ask...)
Rosemary
Jill B.
Sarah G.
Mary S.
Vern P.
Philip J.
Phylis FJ
William W.
Ian P.
Deborah T.
MetaMan Rob
Larry O.
Charles E.
Christine L.
Dr. Robert D.

And all of you that read the e-Alert and let us know how it helped you...moved you...infuriated you...Thank you for your continued support. We literally would not be doing this without you.

Of course, I would be remiss if I didn't thank my "muses"...the FDA, the pharmaceutical giants, the courts (at every level), and the mainstream press and their talent for sensational, misleading headlines.

Let's be honest...they're really the ones that keep it interesting.

Introduction

When I started writing the HSI e-Alert five years ago, I never thought I would find something to write about every day. After all, it's health. It isn't the stock market or Hollywood, where something juicy changes every day.

It turns out I couldn't have been more wrong. Not only do I find something to write about every day, I usually find myself having to set things aside. Beyond having too much information to cover, anyone who knows me knows that I've never had an opinion I didn't feel the need to express. For those two reasons, the HSI e-Alert was expanded to include "And Another Thing."

"And Another Thing" has been the place I've been able to talk about executives for a giant drug company that have been caught doing something unscrupulous, or some elected official who has mounted a campaign to ban a perfectly safe herbal supplement, or an FDA whistleblower who has revealed yet another hidden agenda within that densely layered bureaucracy.

I could go on and on. Actually...I do go on and on. And you're holding the result in your hands.

For this volume I've picked some of my favorite e-Alerts that mostly fall into that "and another thing" category. Between these covers you'll find...

- The truth about what's really contained in commercial milk (and how to avoid it without giving up milk products)

- How the overuse of antibiotics has created superbugs that resist modern medicine's best efforts to kill them (and yes, there are several natural alternatives that kill bacteria without contributing to antibiotic resistance)

- The placebo myth (those "inert" sugar pills used in clinical trials often contain much more than a pinch of sugar)

- The surprising techniques used by drug company salespeople to manipulate doctors (and that manipulation is often more than welcome)

- How the medical mainstream jumped through hoops to put a positive spin on study after study that revealed the grave dangers of synthetic hormone replacement therapy to address menopausal problems (all the while, of course, effective natural therapies have been available...without the dire side effects)

- The way food industries influence the USDA to produce dietary recommendations that don't coincide with principles of good nutrition (I found an alternative Food Pyramid that turns the USDA Pyramid on its head)

- How the subsidiary of a well known drug company knowingly sold contaminated blood plasma overseas (and nearly got away with it)

- How a medical board revoked the license of a brilliant osteopathic doctor for using alternative medicine techniques (even though NONE of his patients had filed a single complaint)

And that's just for starters.

If you're a long-time e-Alert reader I think you may find fresh insights while revisiting these favorite pieces. And if you're new to the e-Alert or this is the first you've ever heard of it, then it's good to have you aboard. But here's fair warning: If these injustices and (sometimes hilarious) misdeeds set your blood boiling, well, brace yourself...because there are many more "and another things" emerging every day.

To Your Good Health,

Jenny Thompson

Jenny Thompson

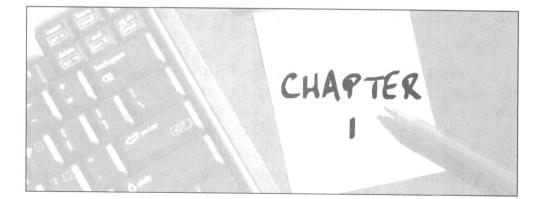

Drug company's greed risks lives of cancer patients

First ran 7/6/2001

As I sipped my morning coffee over the paper two Sundays ago, I suddenly couldn't believe what I was reading. The front page of the "Baltimore Sun" had a shocking headline, "How a cancer trial ended in betrayal." While these events occurred over the past six years, the information was revealed only recently —and by accident. The details of this story, and what we've uncovered since is truly shocking…

Imagine if you had a rare form of skin cancer and volunteered for a drug trial to test a revolutionary product that would "probably" cure your cancer. After just 8 short weeks, the researchers told you that your cancer was virtually cured.

Now imagine it was a lie.

As reported in the Sun, that's what happened to 22 cancer patients who were the innocent victims of a scheme to drive up the stock price of BioCryst Pharmaceuticals. The researchers' primary motivation was getting FDA approval for their drug so their corporate stock would skyrocket. Greed replaced sound practices. Personal gain was the top priority.

To guarantee a good showing for their drug, BioCryst assigned a nurse to "help" with the study: the wife of the scientist who was running the study for the company. She was also a major stockholder and stood to make a great deal of money if the drug received FDA approval. The drug trial was conducted at the University of Alabama, and the chairman of the school's dermatology department became a "consultant" for the drug trial.

And so began the "shell game."

With each passing week, patients' skin lesions were measured to determine growth or reduction. Even though it was obvious to anyone looking that most of the lesions were not disappearing or even getting better, patients were told they were being cured. Since external appearance is just one method of determining remission or cure, the cancer patients were convinced the scientists knew what they were doing and the cancer really was being cured. After all, who would know better than the experts?

At the end of the 8-week drug trial, BioCryst reported to the FDA that 59% of the patients had reduced or eliminated cancer. They'd finally found a cure!

BioCryst's stock soared, going from $6 a share to almost $13 within a few months, and they became the darlings of Wall Street.

The drug company's house of cards tumbled when a company researcher not privy to the plot recalculated the results of the drug trial six months after it ended. He found that only 30% of drug-treated lesions improved. The rate of cure wasn't even close to the 59% reported to the FDA.

What's more, those in the placebo group had results twice as good as those using the "miracle" cream!

When the real results reached the FDA, they launched an investigation. But that didn't help the 22 cancer patients. They had wasted time—and maybe their lives—using a cream that would let their cancers flourish.

This is not a simple case of conflict of interest. It's a case of calculated deceit, corruption, and fraud. BioCryst officials were sentenced to jail and fined (they're appealing their convictions). That's little comfort to the 22 people who had their hopes dashed by greedy conspirators who think that profits are more important than life.

None of this would have come to light—and the 22 cancer victims would never have known they were using a useless cream—if Dr. William Cook, BioCryst's medical director, hadn't been given the real results by mistake. Dr. Cook was writing a scientific article about the drug trial, and he noticed that the results reported to the FDA were not the same (or as bad) as the ones he had. When he asked for other corroborating documents, which were kept in a locked cabinet, he was mistakenly given the actual test data. Until then, no one had been provided the correct data that showed the cream was ineffective.

Even with the poor showing, BioCryst isn't giving up on their cream. While the company's stock sits at $6.45 today, they're continuing to test it, although things don't look any better. In a randomized, double-blind, placebo-controlled study conducted at the prestigious M.D. Anderson Cancer Center in Houston, the topical drug had a 28% success rate in treating skin cancer, while the placebo showed a 24% reduction in skin lesions.

The new "academic-industrial complex" that combines university resources with drug company research dollars has forever changed the face of research.

To Your Good Health,

Jenny Thompson·
Health Sciences Institute

Sources:

- Baltimore Sun, June 24, 2001: "How a cancer trial ended in betrayal"
  J Am Acad Dermatol, 44(6):940-7, 2001

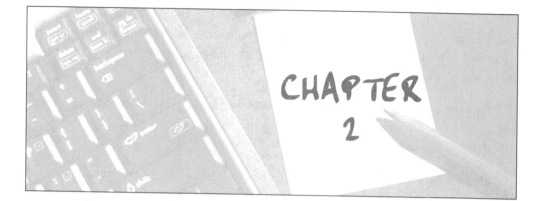

Consumer Reports dons the milk mustache

First ran 8/7/2001

About a year ago, my husband and I bought a house. Our first housewarming gift was from my mother-a subscription to Consumer Reports. And it wasn't too long before it became the most useful gift we got. Within a few months of moving in, the dryer decided it had had it. Soon after, the dishwasher joined its fluff-n-fold friend.

So we pulled out the Consumer Reports and looked for the brand that best suited our needs. (Well, actually, my needs. My husband "needs" either the most expensive model or the one with the most "space-age" features.)

So far, in at least four out of five major purchases in the past year, we deferred to Consumer Reports. Like many of you, the consumer in me has long thought of them as a hype-free zone-exposing the good, the bad and the ugly—to help us make more informed shopping decisions.

However, when I began reading the September issue, I did a double-take when I got to page 62. After reading which SUV in the big-mid-small class they recommend, I was floored:

What on earth are they doing writing an article about whether or not milk "does a body good"? It's one thing to look to them to compare brands of air conditioners, but since when do we turn to them for serious dietary recommendations?

In a two-page "point-counterpoint"-style article, the magazine "evaluates" the health pros and cons of milk.

Throughout the article, Consumer Reports quotes doctors and scientists or their own consultants on the benefits of milk. At the same time, it refers to the controversial animal-rights group People for the Ethical Treatment of Animals (PETA) and the Physicians Committee for Responsible Medicine (PCRM) as "Milk's Critics," offering little research or evidence to back up their points.

Conveniently, it seems any evidence that points against the benefits of milk can be easily explained away.

In one particularly telling paragraph the results of a 12-year, 80,000-participant study conducted by Harvard were completely discounted. According to the study, high milk intake appeared to actually increase the risk of bone fractures among 80,000 nurses. So how does the article explain this proof that milk may actually be bad for your bones? They turn to the lead author of the study, Diane Feskanich, Sc.D., who believes, "...the reason may lie in the nurses' family histories. It may be that those who drank the most milk did so because they faced the highest risk-'but it was too little, too late.'"

But, did Consumer Reports explain how the researcher could so quickly dismiss the results of such an expansive study? Can they really be written off so easily?

The same happened when they reported on two large-scale studies from Harvard that indicate a link between milk consumption and prostate cancer. Though both studies mentioned showed an increase in cancer for those who drank milk, the magazine concludes: "Overall, however, the evidence has been inconsistent, with several studies failing to support that association." (Note that they didn't actually name those studies.)

Other concerns are quickly dismissed, as well. Those of you with colicky children or grandchildren, take comfort. According to the article, if an infant has a milk allergy he will likely outgrow it by age three. Try to hold on until then.

The authors even go so far as to recommend a strategy for lactose-intolerant individuals to reintroduce dairy into their diets!

Despite the heavily slanted treatment in the Consumer Reports article, there's mounting evidence that milk may lead to numerous serious health problems, including cancer, rheumatoid arthritis, atherosclerosis, anemia, MS, leukemia...the list goes on.

And, as the 80,000-nurse-study shows, milk isn't a particularly good source of calcium for those hoping to stave off osteoporosis. In fact, a study published more than a decade ago showed that women who drank three glasses of milk a day lost bone mass at twice the rate of the control group.

As for whether or not you should drink milk...this issue deserves much more than two pages in a magazine designed to tell you which trash bag will hold the most.

The majority of studies we've seen indicate that milk is not the health food the dairy industry would have you believe. Most, if not all, of the doctors and researchers in our network agree that, at the very least, the milk readily available at your local store presents more risks than benefits, as it is laden with hormones and steroids.

If you choose to drink milk, we at Health Sciences Institute recommend you buy only milk from organic dairy farms. But the decision on whether to include dairy in your diet should be one you make after reviewing all the research and talking to your doctor, not one that should be influenced by propaganda and cute marketing slogans.

To Your Good Health,

Jenny Thompson
Health Sciences Institute

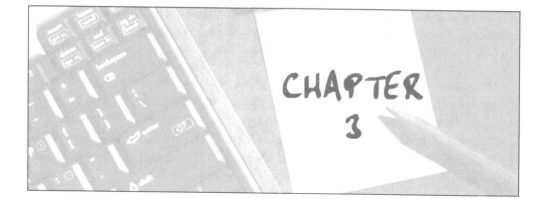

Researchers finally uncover possible links to pancreatic cancer

First ran 8/29/2001

Unfortunately, many, if not all, of us have been through the horror, whether ourselves or with someone we love...a lump in the breast, a swelling of the prostate, or some other symptom that could mean cancer.

Through education and advancements in conventional and alternative medicine, early detection and new treatment options have been able to greatly improve survival rates for many when it is cancer.

This hasn't been the case for pancreatic cancer, however. There are no early warning signs, and according to the National Cancer Institute it has the "poorest likelihood of survival among all major [cancers]." In fact, it's estimated that this year alone about 29,200 cases will be diagnosed, while 28,900 people will die from it.

The American Cancer Society explains that because of the size and location of the pancreas, it is one of the most difficult cancers to detect. The pancreas is a 6-inch-long fish-shaped organ that sits behind your stomach, surrounded by the small intestine. It has two main purposes: 1) it produces the digestive enzymes that break down food and 2) it's the source of hormones (insulin and glucagon) that are important in controlling the amount of sugar in the blood.

While smoking is the single greatest risk factor (accounting for 25-30% of all pancreatic cancer cases), the majority of risk factors identified have been outside of the patient's control—things like age, height, and ethnic group. Two recent studies, however, offer some hope for prevention by identifying two more possible risk factors that can be addressed.

As reported in the August 22nd issue of the Journal of the American Medical Association, researchers at Harvard found a strong link between obesity and pancreatic cancer. They examined the data of over 165,000 subjects for 10 to 20 years. In that period of time, 350 of the patients developed pancreatic cancer.

When the researchers looked more closely, they noticed that the subjects who were clinically obese (or close to it) had a 72 percent higher risk for pancreatic cancer than those who were not obese.

At this stage, researchers aren't sure why this link exists. Nevertheless, the authors of the study make some recommendations. First and most obvious, losing weight will lower your risk of contracting cancer of the pancreas. But exercise seems to diminish the danger, as well. The patients who were obese but active had a risk 41 percent lower than those who were obese and inactive. (Here active is defined as two hours or more of moderate exercise per week.)

The other recent study was published in June by the Journal of the National Cancer Institute. It found a strong association between pancreatic cancer and H. pylori (Helicobacter pylori). H. pylori is a bacterium that has been proven to be the cause of peptic ulcer in the majority of cases.

Participants of the study were drawn from the 29,133 male smokers living in Finland, aged 50 to 69, who participated in a trial called the Alpha-Tocopherol Beta-Carotene (ATBC) Cancer Prevention Study. As smoking is the most consistent risk factor for pancreatic cancer, a larger number of subjects developed pancreatic cancer in the ATBC study than in most other study populations.

The authors of the study compared the levels of antibodies to H. pylori from blood samples taken at the start of the study (before cancer was diagnosed). They compared a group of 121 men who developed pancreatic cancer to a subgroup of 226 men who did not develop cancer but were similar in age and other characteristics.

They found that those infected with certain strains of H. pylori (CagA+) had a two-fold increase in risk of developing pancreatic cancer over the men in the study who were not infected with the bacteria. This study follows another, much smaller study, published in 1998, that also showed a link.

Much more research is necessary to fully evaluate the relationship between H. pylori and pancreatic cancer, particularly since all of those in this study were known to participate in the greatest risk factor—smoking. However, as a result of these studies, researchers are beginning to investigate further how gastric hormones or other factors influenced by H. pylori may affect pancreatic cells. We will be sure to alert you to any future discoveries.

Actions to take:

According to the American Cancer Society, common symptoms of pancreatic cancer include weight loss; abdominal or back pain; loss of appetite; jaundice; digestive problems; stool that is pale, bulky or greasy, blood clots; and diabetes. Should you find you or a loved one are experiencing these symptoms, please consult your doctor immediately.

While there still is no instrument for early detection of pancreatic cancer, we now have some promising research on prevention. Quitting smoking is the most helpful thing you can do, along with controlling your weight and exercising.

We will continue to watch the research on this aggressive cancer and alert you about any further preventive measures or possible alternative treatments.

To Your Good Health,

Jenny Thompson
Health Sciences Institute

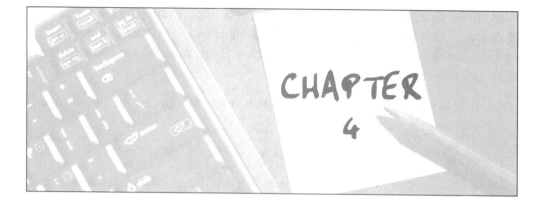

Is the media swimming around the real threat to your health?

First ran 9/05/2001

Nearly three decades ago, an undercurrent of fear was felt through the nation. "Jaws" was in theatres and, thanks to what were amazing special effects at the time, it seemed too real to ignore. I even remember reports about how empty the beaches were.

This summer, the threat has resurfaced, but this time, it's for real. You can't turn on the TV these days or read the paper without hearing about the deadly danger of a shark attack. This morning The Today Show reported that there have been 41 shark attacks in the U.S. this year...three of which were fatal.

And people all seem baffled, assuming there is some mysterious reason that the sharks are suddenly out to get us. They're calling in experts to talk about feeding and swimming patterns, looking at how far they are from shore, what time of day they appear, etc.

But is this really a new phenomenon? Or, is it just that the media has decided to make it this year's summer blockbuster?

I can't help but wonder...

First, consider this surprising bit of information: The number of attacks is deemed by experts to be completely normal for the season, and it's actually down from last year.

Now consider this: So far this summer, there have been 41 shark attacks in the U.S. from which 3 people died. Yet, 31 people have died in the U.S. taking the statin drug Baycol—10 times more than have died in these shark attacks.

So, while people are fleeing the beaches once again, countless patients are still taking statin drugs (among other types of cholesterol-lowering drugs) everyday—potentially risking their lives. But have you heard Katie Couric warning us about that every morning? I haven't heard a second mention in the popular press since I first heard the story on a cable news show a few weeks ago.

And that's not all. While Katie, Matt and the rest of the mainstream media are effectively ignoring the statin story, the pharmaceutical companies' PR machines are working overtime to keep people believing the drugs are safe. Since Bayer pulled Baycol voluntarily, as we reported in the August 9th e-Alert, Bristol-Myers Squibb took out full-page ads in the New York Times, USA Today, and the Philadelphia Inquirer offering a free one-month supply of their drug, Pravachol. Likewise, pharmaceutical giant Merck ran a full-page ad in the Wall Street Journal wooing former Baycol users over to their drug, Zocor.

Talk about sharks circling...

But that's to be expected from the big drug companies. Why the imbalance in news coverage?

One theory, of course, is ratings. The shock value and human-interest focus of the shark attacks is much "sexier" by TV standards than the risk of death by a cholesterol-lowering drug.

But that's only part of it. The other part is the bottom line. Imagine if Bayer had a nationwide aspirin commercial scheduled to run during the Evening News at a price of...let's just say $300,000. Now imagine their marketing director's reaction if the lead story were the number of deaths caused by Baycol. Do you think they would pay that bill? At the very least, I'd think they'd take their millions in advertising dollars elsewhere.

The mainstream media outlets can't afford to bite the hand that's feeding them...so too often important stories like these are either ignored or downplayed.

Now I'm not saying that no one has covered the on-going saga. But the concentration has been terribly weak and the fact that other companies are continuing to aggressively push their statin drugs as substitutes has been completely ignored.

That's one reason we're so pleased we've been able to bring you this free e-Alert service. It allows us to talk to you about issues that the media are ignoring but that we wouldn't normally cover in your monthly Members Alert (or that wouldn't be as timely once you received it).

In recent e-Alerts we've told you about tocotrienol vitamin E, a natural, safe alternative to help manage your cholesterol level. Please make sure you pass on this information regarding the dangers associated with statin drugs and other cholesterol-lowering drugs to any friends or family members you think may be at risk.

To Your Good Health,

Jenny Thompson
Health Sciences Institute

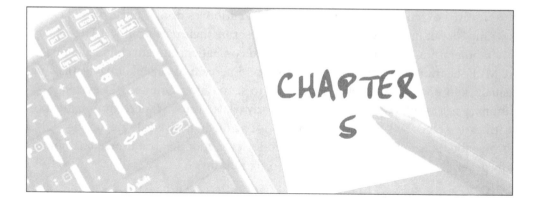

Search for cancer killer leads researchers back to nature

First ran 9/07/2001

It was heralded as possibly the most powerful cancer drug ever developed. Less than three years after testing the first dose on a human (half the normal testing time for a cancer drug), Novartis Pharmaceuticals presented GleevecTM to the FDA for approval. After a short two-and-a-half month review, FDA officials granted the New Drug Application in May. Twenty-four hours after that, trucks loaded with Gleevec pulled out of Novartis's warehouse in East Hanover, New Jersey. Novartis boasts that Gleevec enjoyed the fastest time to market of any cancer treatment in American history.

Novartis executives used phrases like "revolutionary drug," "unsurpassed efficacy," and "breakthrough cancer therapy" to describe their new product. The chemotherapy agent was specially tailored to combat chronic myeloid leukemia (CML)—a strain of cancer that accounts for 15 percent of all leukemia deaths and usually kills end-stage patients within two to six months. Granted, Gleevec's preliminary test results were impressive. In early trials, nearly 90 percent of patients with early-stage CML went into remission. The median survival rate among end-stage patients who tried Gleevec, climbed to seven months (traditional chemotherapy generally lets a patient survive two to six months).

And Gleevec improved the quality of CML sufferers' lives. Novartis acknowledged that the majority of patients treated with Gleevec experienced adverse affects. But unlike standard chemotherapy which assaults the entire immune system, Gleevec targets only the over-active protein that causes CML. Consequently, Gleevec patients suffered notably fewer side-effects than chemo patients.

Enthusiasm for Gleevec soared in the medical community. In the journal Nature, Junia Melo who works on CML at the Imperial College School of Medicine in London, England, said Gleevec's initial success was so impressive that it left some CML researchers wondering if their careers were over. "It's the first designer drug for cancer that's a winner," Melo said.

But just a few short weeks after the FDA approved Gleevec, researchers discovered the drug didn't entirely live up to expectations. In fact, the cancer patients who needed it the most—those with advanced CML—were the ones shortchanged. Scientists at the Molecular Biology Institute at UCLA discovered many patients initially responded to the drug, but then relapsed and grew resistant to Gleevec. Lead researcher Charles Sawyer, M.D., explained that the protein at the root of CML actually fought back against the drug. In some cases, the protein's genetic makeup mutated and rendered the drug useless.

The journal Nature announced the disappointing findings with the headline "Cancer outwits us again."

The problem is that cancer—and a host of other diseases—have been outwitting pharmaceutical companies for ages. And it's not surprising. Pharmaceutical companies have set themselves the daunting challenge of trying to extract some miniscule component from nature; re-engineer, alter, fuse and strengthen it; then dispatch it to fix another incredibly complex product of nature—the human body.

The devil, as they say, is in the details. And in the pharmaceutical process, the number of details—and, hence, the number of opportunities for mistake—is infinite.

One thing that natural—and even some conventional—medicine has shown is that health-protecting substances drawn from nature work best when they're allowed to function the same way they function in their natural state. Remove the 'active ingredient' from an herb and often that ingredient won't produce the same effect. The frustrating truth is that substances don't work in isolation (a situation that regularly foils our efforts to dissect, extract and control nature). Other components typically boost or expand the medicinal value of a natural substance.

You'll see one example of this phenomenon in the October issue of the HSI Members Alert. It's the story of ellagitannin, a substance found in raspberries, walnuts, strawberries, pomegranates, and other fruit. In several published studies, ellagitannin has demonstrated an ability to prevent the growth of cancerous cells and even destroy existing cancer cells. But, as I explained above, ellagitannin works best when you leave it in its natural state.

In tests, Daniel W. Nixon M.D. of the Hollings Cancer Center in South Carolina discovered that the way to get the maximum benefit from this cancer-fighting substance was to pick up some Meeker red raspberries at the market, drop them into a blender, and enjoy the fruit puree. Ellagitannin, extracted from the raspberries, still showed remarkable cancer-fighting abilities. (In one test, cervical cancer cells treated with ellagitannin began to die off with 72 hours.) But the entire raspberry proved even more powerful than the isolated substance. Researchers concluded that other components of the raspberry heightened the effect, but to date, they haven't been able to identify those components or decipher the interaction.

We aren't suggesting that ellagitannin is an absolute cure for cancer. If something as simple as a raspberry could cure cancer, the world never would have known its first oncologist. Further, ellagitannin hasn't yet shown the power to combat a cancer as aggressive as end-stage CML. But the research we've uncovered indicates that it may bolster your natural defenses against developing cancers. And that bolstered immune system can prevent a cell mutation from developing into a malignancy.

HSI Panelist Jon Barron brought the story of ellagitannin to our attention. Working with Healing America, he has developed a supplement made exclusively from the Meeker red raspberries featured in Dr. Nixon's study. Right now, Healing America's supply is limited. That is why we are offering e-Alert members this early opportunity to try this promising treatment.

To learn more about ellagitannin, or to try it out for yourself, follow this link to Healing America's website: http://www.northernnutrition.healingamerica.com.

To Your Good Health,

Jenny Thompson
Health Sciences Institute

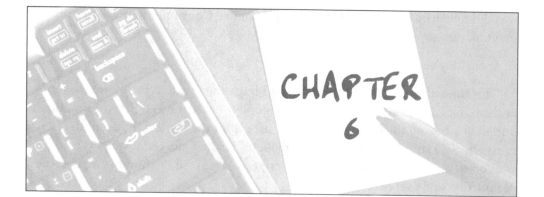

Should HSI start rating appliances?

First ran 9/25/2001

Doo-doo-doo-doo, doo-doo-doo-doo.

That's the theme music from "The Twilight Zone," for those of you following along at home. And I swear it's what I heard yesterday when I thumbed through the October issue of Consumer Reports.

You may remember my rant against Consumer Reports last month. The magazine, which specializes in rating appliances, cars, and household products, devoted several pages to the pros and cons (but mostly the pros) of drinking milk. Besides the fact that the article was incredibly slanted to the pro-milk camp, I thought it was outrageously inappropriate for a magazine like Consumer Reports to comment on the issue at all.

Well, they've done it again.

This time, the topic is diabetes. And although the article is positioned as an evaluation of 11 of the best-selling home blood-glucose meters, that information is buried in a box on the last page. No, the real gist of the story is to "detail the latest, most effective strategies for managing diabetes beyond glucose testing." The piece goes on to push new classes of oral prescription drugs, while minimizing the role of nutrition and exercise.

What is going on here? Since when is Consumer Reports a source of health information? And even more importantly, where are they getting their information? Their recommendations certainly fly in the face of everything we know about Type II diabetes.

Take, for instance, the study that just appeared in the New England Journal of Medicine. It showed that even people at high risk for Type II diabetes could virtually eliminate their risk by changing their eating habits, exercising, and losing weight. That study followed 522 people for four years. All of the participants were in the classic risk group: 40-65 years old, overweight (BMIs of 25 or higher), and already exhibiting glucose intolerance, a precursor to Type II diabetes. Half of them were assigned to a control group, and told to go about their normal habits. The other half attended sessions on nutrition and exercise, and were asked to work toward five goals: reducing weight by five percent or more, reducing total fat intake to less than 30 percent of total energy, reducing saturated fat intake to less than 10 percent of total energy consumed, increase fiber intake to at least 15 grams per 1,000 calories, and exercise 30 minutes a day or more.

Here's the amazing result: not one of the participants who achieved at least four of the five goals developed diabetes—not even after four years! Even those who were only able to reach some of the goals cut their incidence rate by 58 percent over the control group.

This isn't the only study that shows diet and lifestyle can successfully treat Type II diabetes. Yet the Consumer Reports story made no mention of these findings. In fact, the story reported, "People with diabetes no longer need to follow a specialized diet plan."

Here's another nice spin from the article: "Lifestyle changes can control the glucose level in some cases. But most [Type II diabetes] patients also need oral drugs; many will eventually need insulin shots, too." Here's another one: "Most people with Type II diabetes need medication to control their glucose level...Most diabetes patients should probably be taking more than one medication." How thoughtful of the editor to also include a chart listing four new types of oral drugs that "attack Type II diabetes from different angles." The more I read, the more it seemed like a press release from a pharmaceutical company.

The bizarreness of it all heightened as I read the last page, where they finally get around to talking about the blood-glucose meters diabetics use. Like a kid looking at a holiday catalog of new toys, they described the bells and whistles on the various meters, and new gadgets that may eliminate the need for diabetics to routinely stick themselves with needles to monitor glucose levels.

I can understand their excitement. Authorities tell us that some 10 million Americans have been diagnosed with diabetes, and another five million diabetics may be undiagnosed. In the next 25 years, they expect those numbers to double. That's a whole lot of potential consumers for a whole new world of gadgets and drugs.

But nowhere along the way does the author stop and ask "Why?" Why are more and more people being diagnosed with Type II diabetes every year? Why is a disease that used to be associated with the elderly now being seen in adolescents and even children?

Truthfully, I don't want Consumer Reports asking those questions. But someone should. Conventional authorities have scratched the surface and offered some theories—among them our nation's increasing rate of obesity, our high intake of refined carbohydrates, and our overall sedentary lifestyle. But we need to know more, and the messages need to be communicated more effectively to the general public. And it certainly shouldn't come from publications like Consumer Reports, in a thinly veiled attempt to promote new band-aid drugs and devices.

At HSI, we've been devoted to bringing you breakthrough health information for over five years. And along the way, we've told you about several natural approaches to help control your blood glucose levels. In the March 2001 issue, we told you about Normalose, the herbal tea extract that can lower blood sugar levels by 32 percent in just three weeks. The May 2000 issue covered UltraGlycemX, a nutrient-rich beverage that helps improve insulin-response and serum glucose levels. We'll continue to track new discoveries about Type II diabetes, and bring you real information you can use.

That's as it should be—because that's why we come to work each day. It's our whole reason for publishing. And we intend to stick to that. Consumer Reports may have revised their mission statement, but don't worry—you won't see us rating refrigerators any time soon.

To Your Good Health,

Jenny Thompson
Health Sciences Institute

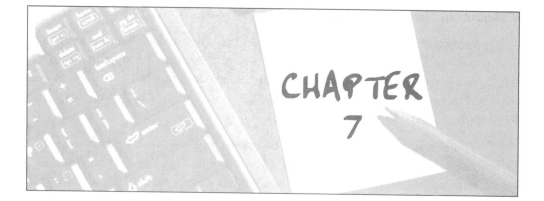

Could your arthritis cure put you at risk for heart attack?

First ran 10/8/2001

Lies of omission. That's what my mother calls them.

The kind where you provide small amounts of information strictly on a "need-to-know" basis. I never considered it lying—just not telling the whole truth. If someone didn't get the pertinent information—that was their own fault. "You didn't ask me THAT," used to be my defense when I got caught in one of my webs. And, yes, inevitably—I always got caught.

Recently, pharmaceutical giant Merck & Co. has gotten caught in a lie of omission over its blockbuster arthritis drug Vioxx—and the company is responding like a 13-year-old caught with a cigarette behind his back.

I'm sure you've seen the commercials for Vioxx. They end with a reminder to "ask you doctor" about this new drug for arthritis. Well, lots of people followed that advice—Vioxx is one of the fastest selling drugs in the world, and sales are expected to reach $2 billion or more by 2002. Not bad for a drug that received FDA approval just a little over a year ago.

But you may not see those Vioxx ads too much longer—or, at least, they won't be quite the same. The FDA has ordered Merck to halt all promotion of Vioxx because the ads minimize the popular drug's safety risks—particularly a startling increased risk of heart attack.

The finding came out in a Merck-sponsored study that first appeared in The New England Journal of Medicine in late 2000. It found that people over 40 with rheumatoid arthritis who took Vioxx had FOUR TIMES the risk of heart attack as comparable people who took naproxen, the NSAID found in over-the-counter painkiller Aleve and other prescription pain medications.

Believe it or not, that little tidbit snuck under the radar for a while. The Merck study was not designed to track the drugs' effects on heart health; it was supposed to demonstrate that Vioxx caused fewer ulcers and other GI problems than naproxen. It accomplished that goal; among the study's 8,076 participants, the people taking Vioxx had about half the incidence of upper GI "events," as compared with those who took naproxen. (Vioxx's active ingredient, rofecoxib, is in a new class of drugs called Cox-2 inhibitors which had been roundly praised for effectively eliminating pain without causing gastrointestinal damage, as NSAIDs like naproxen can do.)

Merck submitted the study to the FDA to help prove that Vioxx should not be required to carry a gastro-intestinal warning on its label. And it proceeded to blanket the public with marketing campaigns touting Vioxx's lower risk of gastro-intestinal problems.

But, eventually, the truth caught up with them. Some doctors and researchers quietly started asking questions about the cardiovascular findings in the Merck study. Finally, the FDA asked Merck about the findings.

Merck claims that the findings only demonstrate the blood-thinning effects of naproxen on cardiovascular health, not that Vioxx actually harms the heart. And, to be fair, their advertisements do reveal that Vioxx does not thin the blood.

But others wonder if there's more to the story. Some doctors and researchers are calling for more research into the possible mechanisms behind the four-fold increase in heart attacks in the Merck study. The FDA noted that there's no proof that the heart attack discrepancy can be completely explained away by naproxen's blood thinning benefits. "In fact, the situation is not at all clear," stated the FDA in its response to Merck.

And then in late September, the FDA issued the cease-and-desist order on Vioxx ads. We don't yet know how Merck will respond—but stay tuned.

Granted, the cardiovascular risk from Vioxx is fairly small—the numbers work out to an increase of four heart attacks per 1,000 patients. But it is still significant, and it joins an already extensive list of warnings, contraindications, precautions, and possible side effects on the Vioxx label.

And remember that Vioxx does nothing to rebuild worn cartilage or address the underlying causes of arthritis. It only helps manage the pain. Why accept the risks associated with it when there are so many safe, natural alternatives for relieving arthritis pain and helping heal damaged joints?

HSI has written about dozens of natural arthritis therapies. In June 2001, we told you about the topical deep-tissue oil "Pain Away," which combines 10 proven painkillers in a formula that blocks the pain message sent to your brain. In July 2000, we covered the Ayurvedic herbal formulas like Boswellia, which has been proven to inhibit the action of the inflammatory agents that lead to joint stiffness and arthritis pain. A recent e-Alert brought you an update on Lyprinol, the natural remedy derived from New Zealand green-lipped mussels. We originally covered Lyprinol in our December 1999 issue, when we first learned about this natural therapy that is proven to inhibit the 5-lipoxygenase pathway, one of the biochemical pathways involved in inflammatory response.

And in our December issue, we'll tell you about another promising arthritis treatment. Currently, we are researching the analgesic properties of JointCare—a formula of several Ayurvedic (Indian) herbs from Himalaya USA. This mixture of extracts from guggul, Indian madder, horseradish tree and five other Indian plants has proven effective in relieving pain caused by rheumatoid arthritis and osteoarthritis. Furthermore, toxicity studies (lasting up to two years) have concluded that the formula doesn't induce adverse side effects. We'll continue our research and bring you full details in December's HSI Members Alert.

Maybe Merck has learned a valuable lesson from this experience: that it's always best to tell the whole story, the first time. But this is not just about Merck—it's the entire pharmaceutical industry, which values profits over people's health. We need to teach others to question their doctors and the advertisements they see on TV, and to make informed choices about their health. You can help by passing this information along to anyone you know who takes Vioxx and make sure they know about all the potential risks they face—not just the ones Merck decided not to omit.

To Your Good Health,

Jenny Thompson
Health Sciences Institute

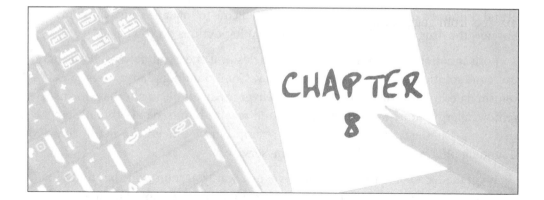

FDA looking for even more control over our health choices

First ran 11/19/2001

Imagine that you had a child with a history of life-threatening allergic reactions. Your child develops a raging infection, which requires treatment with a specific class of antibiotic. The problem is, that antibiotic contains yellow dye #5—a substance that you know would induce a severe reaction in your child. What would you do?

Or, say you suffer from an extremely rare condition that is controlled by a specific prescription drug. But the patent expires, and the pharmaceutical company decides that there isn't enough demand for the drug to justify the expense of a patent renewal and continued production. You need the medicine to manage your symptoms—but now the drug will no longer be available. What options do you have?

Both situations present formidable obstacles. But the good news is, both share the same solution—compounding pharmacy. Compounding pharmacists can reformulate drugs with expired patents, deliver medications in alternate forms, remove allergy-inducing dyes and fillers, and resolve hundreds of other obstacles that can get in the way of following the prescriptions you need. For many, compounding pharmacy provides a life-saving service.

Yet, if the meddlers in Washington have their way, you soon won't be able to FIND a compounding pharmacist—they'll have been regulated right out of business.

Apparently, the FDA doesn't think free speech applies to alternative medicine

In late October, the U.S. Supreme Court agreed to hear a case that will decide if the government can regulate compounding at local pharmacies. Although the case (known as Thompson v. Western States Medical Center, 01-344) won't reach the Supreme Court until 2002, its roots reach back to 1997. That's when Congress passed the Food and Drug Administration Modernization Act (FDAMA), which, among other things, restricted compounders' abilities to advertise their services and wares. Pharmacies in Nevada filed suit against the federal government, charging that the restrictions violated the free speech clause of the First Amendment. A federal appeals court agreed with them, and went one step further, saying the entire compounding section of the FDAMA was unconstitutional. Now the FDA has appealed that decision to the Supreme Court.

According to a report by the Associated Press, the Bush administration urged the court to take the case, "arguing that there were serious health implications in allowing unregulated drug-mixing." In one communication, the AP says Bush administration officials told the Supreme Court that unrestricted compounding "would seriously impair the integrity of the drug approval process."

Excuse me, but could someone please show me the so-called "integrity" in the drug approval process? I guess I haven't been paying close enough attention. And what exactly are these "serious health implications"? Tell that to the thousands of people who depend on compounding to AVOID the serious health implications of mass-produced commercial drugs.

What all this really comes down to is money. The FDA and pharmaceutical companies are afraid of compounding because they can't control it—which means they can't profit from it.

You see, compounding pharmacists don't just count out and measure mass-produced drugs as most pharmacists do. Compounders work with your doctor to create a medicine that best fits your specific needs. Ingredients, dosage, concentration, delivery method, flavoring—all of these variables are within the control of the prescribing physician and compounder. For example, a compounding pharmacist can combine two medications into one pill, or formulate some medications into lotions, eye drops, lip balms, nebulizer solutions, or suppositories. They give you options where you thought there were none.

It's not just a matter of convenience—in many cases, compounding comes to the rescue in life-threatening situations. For instance, many critically ill patients in hospice care rely on compounded medications because they are unable to swallow pills. I'd like to see the FDA talk to them about "serious health implications."

Pharmacists are professionals—
let's treat them that way

We're not talking about any old Joe playing mad scientist with a bunch of controlled substances. We're talking about licensed, educated pharmacists with years of training. They cannot dispense any medications, compounded or otherwise, without a doctor's prescription. In fact, doctors are the ones who usually initiate the compounding order, asking the pharmacists to formulate the medication according to his or her specifications. All of the ingredients are approved drugs listed in the U.S. Pharmacopoeia National Formulary (USP/NF), an encyclopedia of all drugs approved by the U.S. Pharmaceutical Convention. There's plenty of regulation here already (and I mean plenty). So let's let pharmacists be pharmacists, not just glorified pill-counters.

From listening to the FDA, you'd think that there were compounders on every corner. But the truth is, the use of compounding is not that wide spread. Many people are still not aware of compounding, and those who are aware often have difficulty finding a compounding pharmacist in their area, or a doctor who is comfortable working with one. With such a low profile, it hardly poses a threat to the billion-dollar-a-year pharmaceutical industry. The few dollars they may lose to compounding is certainly no reason to eliminate a powerful alternative that offers so much help to so many.

At HSI, we've done our best to spread the word. Our members will remember our in-depth coverage of compounding pharmacy in the May 2000 issue of the Members Alert newsletter. If you'd like to find a compounding pharmacist in your area, go to the International Academy of Compounding Pharmacists' website at iacprx.org, where you'll also find additional information for you AND your doctor on the benefits of compounding.

There's nothing we can do to influence the Supreme Court decision. But we can keep up our fight against the forces in Washington that continually seek to limit our choices about our own health. Write to the FDA and tell them that you don't appreciate their vendetta against compounding pharmacy. You can send your message to the FDA from their website, at http://www.fda.gov. You can also write to your senators and representatives in Congress and tell them that you support compounding pharmacy. For an email directory of all the members of the House of Representatives, go to house.gov/writerep; for an email directory of the Senate, go to senate.gov. Finally, forward this message to anyone you think would be concerned about the government taking away their right to work with their own doctor and pharmacist to protect themselves.

We need to let the "powers that be" know that we ARE paying attention—and that we want them to let us make our own choices when it comes to our health care.

To Your Good Health,

Jenny Thompson
Health Sciences Institute

Sources:

- (1) "Court to Consider Drug Mixing Case,"
  Associated Press, October 29, 2001

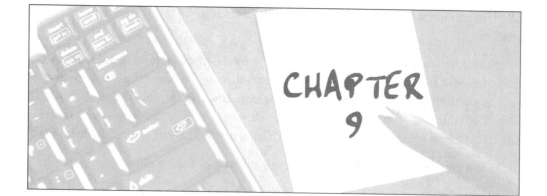

Does Merck's new research prove cholesterol is not the problem?

First ran 11/28/2001

I remember the conversation as if it were yesterday. My friend Wendy called, sobbing uncontrollably. I could hardly understand what she was trying to tell me. Finally, she got the words out. Her father—a seemingly healthy, fit, active man—died from a heart attack. He didn't smoke. He exercised and watched what he ate. He even had low cholesterol. But still—a heart attack took his life.

I knew Wendy's dad as long as I could remember, so his death struck particularly close to home. But it wasn't the first—or unfortunately, the last time I heard a similar story. Every day, heart attacks and strokes kill or disable people who never saw it coming. They thought they were safe—because their cholesterol levels were within "normal" range.

At HSI, we've been writing about this for years. High cholesterol is not a disease in and of itself. Cholesterol does not CAUSE heart disease, it is merely a marker—and one marker out of many. Having "normal" or even low cholesterol levels does not eliminate your risk of heart attack or stroke. Unfortunately, many people who rely on the mainstream (or their doctors) for health information haven't gotten the message.

When you've only got a hammer, every problem looks like a nail.

Maybe the mainstream hasn't focused on the other known markers of heart disease because the pharmaceutical companies haven't come up with a pill to treat them. The focus has been on lowering cholesterol because that's what they're selling—and they're selling plenty. (Statin drugs, the class of cholesterol-lowering drugs that includes Mevacor and Zocor, were one of the top-sellers last year, adding $8.2 billion dollars to the coffers.)

From what I've seen in recent headlines, the statin coffers will continue to grow. Just a few weeks ago, a report presented at the American Heart Association's annual Scientific Sessions meeting proclaimed that even MORE people should be taking cholesterol-lowering drugs. "Cholesterol drug could help millions," proclaimed MSNBC; that's pretty representative of the fawning coverage I saw from most media outlets.

But, as usual, the headlines don't tell the whole story. To me, the report created more questions than answers. Other presentations at the same AHA meeting seemed to supply contradictory information. But the bottom line is that the mainstream's own research is PROVING what we've been saying all along—cholesterol is NOT the main cause of heart disease.

The new approach:
treating a problem that doesn't exist

The AHA's Scientific Sessions were held in mid-November. Doctors and researchers from all over the world presented their findings on the latest research on cardiovascular disease—what causes it, how to treat it, and who is at risk. The presentation that got the most attention was based on data extrapolated from the Oxford Cholesterol Study, which continuously enrolled participants between 1991 and 2001.

Over the course of the study, a total of 20,536 people enrolled, and each was followed for an average of five years. All the participants were between the ages of 40 and 80, and were considered at high-risk for heart attack or stroke. (People with diabetes, a previous heart attack or stroke, and those with artherosclerosis were considered "high-risk.") They were randomly assigned to receive either Merck's statin drug, Zocor, or a placebo. The study recorded any incidence of heart attack, stroke, death from any cause, and vascular procedures like angioplasty and bypass surgery.

This study was the first to show that even "high-risk" people with normal to low cholesterol can slash their risk of heart attack and stroke by taking a statin like Zocor.

"The remarkable thing we found is that cholesterol-lowering therapy benefits all groups of high-risk individuals, irrespective of their cholesterol levels," said Dr. Rory Collins, the lead researcher from University of Oxford in England. "So it didn't matter if a patient's cholesterol level was considered low—we saw the same reduction in risk as people who had the highest levels." Dr. Collins went even farther in an interview with MSNBC. "There is no threshold [of blood cholesterol] below which one should-n't treat these patients," he said. "This really blew us away. It changes everything."

It certainly changes something, though it's not clear what that "something" is. (Some might say it dramatically changes Merck's bottom line, as the new findings could potentially expand their target market by some 160 million people.) The media coverage seemed to ignore the irony, focusing only on the fact that the drugs might be recommended more widely. The public was left with the impression that just about everyone should be taking Zocor. But no one seemed to question the obvious truth that seems to be lying just under the surface.

Think about it: if cholesterol were the main cause of heart disease, as the mainstream touts, why would a person who starts out with low cholesterol be at "high-risk"? And if they reduce their overall risk by taking statins, what problem is the statin actually addressing? Because it obviously isn't the cholesterol.

It may seem like a leap but couldn't you almost say that Merck's study on Zocor PROVES that cholesterol isn't the main cause of heart disease?

The mainstream can't see the forest through the trees

I'll agree that this study brings us important new data. But I'd say the conclusion is all wrong. Maybe statin drugs can help millions more people. But the really exciting finding here is that it's not because of cholesterol. This study should be a wake-up call to conventional medicine, forcing it to recognize that there are many other factors involved. It should trigger a flood of new studies, intent on naming the other markers that influence heart disease risk, and how statins work—or don't work—against them.

At HSI, we've written about the many other theories and causes of heart disease, as well as various other markers that can signal an increased risk of heart attack or stroke. Some of the topics included high homocysteine levels (March 2000 Members Alert newsletter), depleted Coenzyme Q10 stores (September 1999 Members Alert), elevated levels of platelet-activating-factor and thromboxane AZ (November 1999 Members Alert), and high levels of free radicals in the bloodstream that attack artery walls. Each of these markers can be a red flag for heart disease risk—and when all are taken into consideration, in conjunction with total cholesterol and HDL/LDL ration, they can provide much clearer warning signs before it's too late.

This is such an important topic, and there is so much to say, that I can't fit it all in one e-Alert—at least not one you'll continue reading. Tomorrow I'll tell you more about how you can assess heart disease markers beyond cholesterol—and what you can do about it if you find that you are at risk. Until tomorrow...

To Your Good Health,

Jenny Thompson
Health Sciences Institute

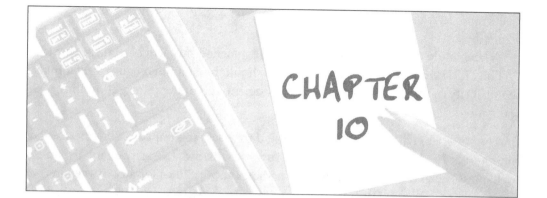

Have you insulted your doctor lately?

First ran 12/14/2001

Cancer patients everywhere can breathe a sigh of relief now that we have proof that doctors aren't insulted when patients look elsewhere for information about their disease.

That's the message from an article I read yesterday on Reuters Health. "Docs Not Insulted When Patients Scour Health News," read the headline. And the story goes on to praise oncologists for patiently tolerating their patients' questions and quests for more information.

Of all the examples of medical egomania and media apathy this may be the worst.

"It's all about ME!"

When you look at the actual research that spawned this article, you see that PATIENTS are the real story. The big news should be that oncologists are failing the majority of their patients by not providing enough of the information they want and deserve.

The study I'm talking about was designed to assess the impact of the media and the Internet on the treatment of cancer. To gather their data, researchers distributed questionnaires in the lobbies of Canadian cancer clinics for a two-week period. They also mailed questionnaires to all doctors registered with Canadian oncology associations. The cancer patients were asked questions about their sources of health information, how they were coping with their illness, and basic demographic information. The doctors were asked their opinions of medical information in the media and on the Internet, and the impact this information has on their patients and practices. A total of 191 cancer patients and 410 oncologists completed the questionnaires and were included in the analysis.

Here's what they found: most cancer patients (86.4 percent) said they wanted "as much information as possible about their illness." Yet the majority of those patients (53.7 percent) said the information they received from their physicians and other health care providers was "insufficient."

Don't let the door hit you on the way out of the doctor's office...

When you look at the rest of the data, that's not surprising. The majority of oncologists (54.2 percent) reported spending less than 15 minutes with their patients during office visits. Another big chunk (36.2 percent) reported spending between 15 minutes and 30 minutes. That leaves fewer than 40 doctors out of more than 400 who reported spending more than 30 minutes with patients on a regular basis. And remember, these are cancer patients, not people with sore throats.

According to Dr. Lillian Siu, an oncologist and one of the lead researchers in the study, "Physicians in a busy practice can't give them [cancer patients] as much information as they would like to obtain...the time we have to answer the extra questions isn't always feasible." I understand the point...but if doctors can't give cancer patients their full time and attention, exactly whom are they saving it for?

As the headline was quick to point out, most doctors reported feeling "neutral" (45.3 percent) or "supportive" (38.4 percent) about their patients who search for additional medical information. (Another 16 percent reported feeling "mildly irritated.") Yet I noticed that patients weren't asked how they felt about their doctors' inability to provide them with enough information. Considering that many of the patients surveyed have spent more than 30 hours searching for information their doctors couldn't give them, you'd think some of them might feel "mildly irritated," too.

Here's the bottom line: patients have the right and the responsibility to take charge of their health. If doctors don't like it, too bad. We shouldn't be asking doctors how patients can make things easier for them—doctors should be focusing on ways to serve patients' needs. We need to change the way we think about health care, and put patients where they belong—in the center.

If your doctor doesn't give you enough time and attention, demand more. If you feel that your doctor is irritated by your knowledge of health issues, find a new doctor. I know it's not always that easy, but it's the only way we'll change the status quo. At the very least, have an open discussion with your doctor about your concerns, and make it clear that you expect an open dialogue about health information you bring to the table—not a condescending pat on the head.

As for us, we'll keep bringing you the latest breakthrough health information to help you make your own choices and continue learning about all the options. Even if your doctor might get "mildly irritated" that you know about new research before he does.

To Your Good Health,

Jenny Thompson
Health Sciences Institute

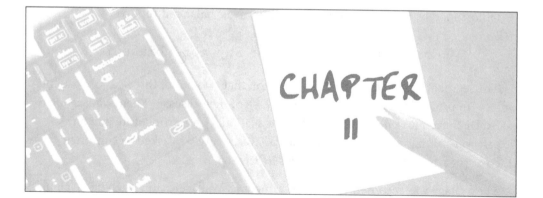

CHAPTER
11

Broadcast highlights mainstream's bias

First ran 1/31/2002

Journalism is supposed to be impartial and unbiased. We all know that it's not. But sometimes the mainstream media's bias is so blatant that I wonder how they've been able to maintain their cloak of neutrality for so long.

I'm talking about last week's news magazine segment on alternative cancer treatments. Chris Wallace from ABC's "Primetime" news magazine clearly enjoyed the role of reporter-turned-spy as he poked around in several clinics in Mexico. It had all the trappings of today's "good television": hidden cameras, awkward confrontations, and doors slamming in faces.

Unfortunately, it didn't have much in the way of balanced reporting.

Could the "experts" be any more biased?

The segment started out with the revelation that two out of three cancer patients will try "unproven" treatment during the course of their disease. Then Wallace introduced Dr. Steven Rosenberg, the head of the National Cancer Institute and an "expert" on "cutting-edge cancer treatments." Rosenberg was asked to comment on a video of visits to several alternative clinics in Tijuana, Mexico.

The footage was recorded via hidden camera as Wallace visited each clinic along with a 75-year-old ovarian cancer patient from California who agreed to cooperate with ABC. In all, the show highlighted three clinics, which offered a variety of alternative cancer therapies like coffee enemas, electromagnetic therapy, insulin-induced coma therapy, ozonation, and hyperbaric chamber therapy. The Mexican video's dramatic conclusion came when the ovarian cancer patient, who had previously undergone unsuccessful treatment at one of the featured clinics, was brought back to confront the clinic's director.

As each therapy was introduced, Rosenberg dismissed them out of hand with terms like "mumbo jumbo." I imagine his expertise in "cutting-edge cancer treatments" involves only those that come with a prescription.

And the entire broadcast zeroed in on the point that the ovarian cancer patient had spent over $15,000 on insulin-induced coma therapy at the clinic, which did nothing to halt the progression of her cancer. Yet no one commented on the fact that chemotherapy and other accepted conventional treatments have done nothing to help her, either. (And you can be sure that she didn't get chemotherapy for free.)

As if the coverage weren't already biased enough, ABC then brought in Dr. Stephen Barrett to comment on alternative medicine. For those of you unfamiliar with Barrett, he is the founder of QuackWatch, a website bent on discrediting alternative medicine. He was presented as an "expert," although is a retired psychiatrist with no particular experience or education in cancer treatment or alternative medicine.

You never know where greatness will come from

The day after the broadcast, Barrett participated in a live chat on alternative therapies on ABC's website. I don't have enough room here to refute all the outrageous, close-minded, ignorant statements he made. But one in particular stood out.

"To my knowledge, there has not been a single idea in the past 50 years that was thought to be quackery and was later demonstrated to be useful," Barrett said.

Really? That's an interesting viewpoint. But I would emphatically disagree.

What about PC-Spes? Immunotherapy? Photodynamic therapy? All of these cancer treatments approaches were once thought of as "alternative." Now they are widely accepted as mainstream.

If we reach beyond the realm of cancer research, I can think of even more. St. John's Wort. Gingko biloba. Garlic. More than a few people called Linus Pauling a quack and he went on to win the Nobel Prize for his work on vitamin C.

And if we go back further than 50 years, there are many more examples of discredited ideas that revolutionized the world. I'm sure plenty of Watson and Crick's colleagues thought they were wasting their time building a big model with little balls—yet look at the amazing strides science has made since they broke the genetic code. And what about that crazy guy who believed the world was round, when everyone knew it was flat?

Don't let THEM control your options

Sure, there are quacks out there—in every branch of medicine, and in many other realms of society as well. We all have to exercise caution, especially when making decisions about our health.

But there's only one person qualified to make those decisions—and that's YOU. I don't want some doctor at the NCI (or heaven forbid, someone like Stephen Barrett) deciding what therapies I can have access to. I want information about the pros and cons of all of my options—and only then will I make the choice that's best for me.

As this broadcast illustrated, the mainstream media is generally not a good source of that information. Here at HSI, we'll continue to try to fill that void, by bringing you the latest breakthrough research on all kinds of medical treatment. And we'll continue to encourage you to find out more about treatment approaches that interest you and apply to your particular condition. There's only one thing we won't do—make those decisions for you. There are enough people out there trying to do that already.

More information about the PrimeTime broadcast, and the chat with Dr. Barrett can be seen on the ABC website, www.abcnews.com.

To Your Good Health,

Jenny Thompson
Health Sciences Institute

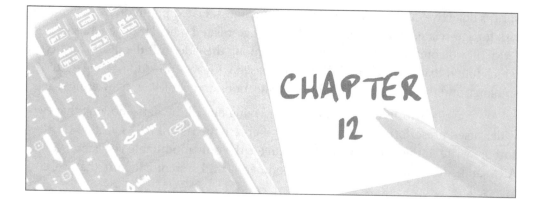

Mainstream's blindness on macular degeneration

First ran 2/20/2002

Here at HSI, our inboxes are always piled high with scientific studies. Everyone on staff shares their findings, as we search for new discoveries to cover in the Members Alert newsletter, or new research to discuss in upcoming e-Alerts. Usually, we share studies that we think are valuable to our members. But occasionally, one of us will come across a study that's noteworthy for a different reason— because its findings are so absurd.

That was the case yesterday, when one of our editors came across a study that appeared in the Archives of Ophthalmology late last year. The abstract states the study's objective: to describe the risk factors and associated population attributable risk for age-related maculopathy (ARM) and age-related macular degeneration (AMD), two common causes of vision loss among the elderly. It details its results, which found that ARM and AMD risk increased with age (no kidding), cigarette smoking, and the use of ACE inhibitor medications and cholesterol-lowering drugs.

Are you ready for the punch line? After laying out all the data showing that two widely used prescription drug classes can increase the risk of ARM and AMD, the authors write in their conclusion: "Smoking is the only modifiable risk factor for ARM and AMD, among the many environmental and systemic factors that were assessed."

Excuse me? Maybe these guys read another study.

Common prescription drugs more dangerous for your eyes than smoking

Let's review the details. The researchers recruited 4,345 people over the age of 40 from both rural and urban areas in Australia. They assessed the eye health of each participant, and asked them questions about their health history, lifetime sunlight exposure, and dietary intake. Then, through statistical analysis, they calculated the relative associations between the different factors and ARM/AMD diagnosis.

The study's authors list the risk factors separately for ARM and AMD, even though they showed many commonalities. Not surprisingly, age was the leading risk factor for both conditions. They also shared the same #2 risk factor, namely, a family history of ARM or AMD and #3, use of the prescription blood pressure drugs called ACE inhibitors. For ARM, use of cholesterol-lowering medication took fourth place—but there was no association found between these drugs and AMD. Finally, way down in fifth (or, at best, fourth) place is cigarette smoking— the "only modifiable risk factor."

No one would argue that you can change your age or your family history. But since when is prescription drug use not modifiable? And we're not talking life-giving drugs like insulin for type I diabetics—we're talking about drugs for high blood pressure and cholesterol, two conditions that are often easily remedied with natural approaches and lifestyle changes.

You CAN change the mainstream's drug habit

The mainstream is so immersed in its own "drug culture" that taking ACE inhibitors and statin drugs seems like the status quo. It doesn't occur to them that there might be another way, that the situation can be changed.

We've written many times about natural therapies for lowering blood pressure and reducing cholesterol so you don't have to resort to ACE inhibitors, like lisinopril (Monopril, Prinivil, Zestril) and perindopril (Aceon), and statin drugs, like lovastatin (Mevacor) and atorvastatin (Lipitor).

We've also written about safe and natural therapies to prevent and slow the progression of AMD, like Astafactor, the powerful antioxidant we wrote about in the November 2001 issue of the Members Alert newsletter. Astafactor contains astaxanthin, a specific antioxidant that can pass the blood-brain barrier. (For more information about Astafactor and to order, call Aquasearch at 1-800-480-6515.)

But there's a bigger issue here—namely, that medical research is not all it's cracked up to be. This isn't the first example of a study published in a major peer-reviewed medical journal that blatantly ignored the obvious. And I'm sure it won't be the last.

We'll keep looking for those breakthrough studies that actually reveal new and innovative ways to address your health concerns. And, we'll keep pointing out studies like these that overlook the facts—and could put your health at risk. If you have ARM or AMD and are taking either ACE inhibitor or statin drugs, they could be making your vision worse. Consider natural alternatives for addressing your high blood pressure and cholesterol and talk to your doctor about weaning you off the drugs.

To Your Good Health,

Jenny Thompson
Health Sciences Institute

P.S. For more on natural approaches to managing your blood pressure and cholesterol, search the HSI website for back issues at www.hsibaltimore.com

Sources:

- Archives of Ophthalmology 2001; 119 (10):1455-1462

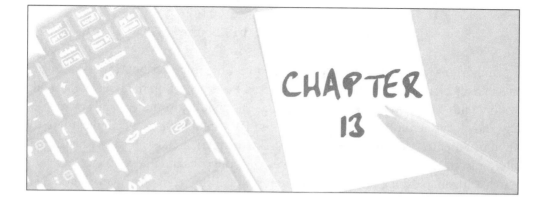

CHAPTER
13

Strange bedfellows: Could a popular RA drug lead to liver damage?

First ran 4/1/2002

When the FDA approved the rheumatoid arthritis drug Arava in 1998, it noted that the new drug wasn't any better than the existing treatments. But, they said, RA patients needed "some different options."

Since then, about 200,000 people have taken the Arava "option." At least 130 people have experienced severe liver toxicity, 56 have been hospitalized, and 12 have died. And an unlikely collection of organizations around the world have called for varying levels of action again this drug—from outright bans to carefully worded physician warnings.

Six times greater risk— but most doctors still unaware

Authorities note that many doctors are continuing to prescribe Arava—because most aren't aware of the risks. In an Associated Press report on the issue, Dr. David Yokum said "I do not believe that the general rheumatologist understands or has any knowledge about these serious and potentially life threatening complications." Yokum, a medical doctor now in private practice in Arizona, is a former scientific advisor to the FDA. Now, he's joined forces with the consumer advocacy group Public Citizen in calling on the FDA to remove the drug from pharmacy shelves.

In a recent press release, the director of Public Citizen's Health Research Group, Dr. Sidney Wolfe, compared the use of Arava (leflunomide) with the use of Rheumatrex (methotrexate), long considered the "gold standard" prescription drug treatment for rheumatoid arthritis. He found that the FDA had received SIX TIMES more reports of liver damage from Arava use as from Rheumatrex use— even though Rheumatrex is taken by thousands more people and has been in use much longer. And as Dr. Yokum noted, "it is impossible to predict which patients will be at risk."

As if a former FDA scientist and Public Citizen aren't strange enough bedfellows, there's more. Early last year, the European Union warned patients and doctors about the drug. And in August, the mainstream even got in on the act: the American College of Rheumatology (ACR) issued a warning about Arava. While the ACR stopped short of calling for a ban, it did advise its member doctors that Arava "should be used with caution."

Damage done in as little as three days

The ACR report also contains more specifics about the drug's risks. In the known cases of serious side effects, most occurred in the first six months of treatment. (In some cases, problems surfaced in as little as three days, while in others, damage appeared after three years of treatment.) It also reported that the liver damage struck indiscriminately across age and gender lines.

But the ACR report does highlight some major risk factors. Most of the Arava users who suffered side effects had also been diagnosed with heart disease, diabetes, or hepatitis. And most were also taking another drug known to cause liver damage at the same time they were taking Arava. The ACR report makes special note of the concomitant use of Arava and nonsteroidal anti-inflammatory drugs (NSAIDs) like ibuprofen (Advil, Motrin), naproxen sodium (Aleve), celecoxib (Celebrex), and rofecoxib (Vioxx), and further warns patients not to drink alcohol while taking Arava.

The ACR also cautions against the experimental approach of combining Arava and Rheumatrex for the treatment of RA. Earlier research had shown that a combination of both drugs could be more effective than either alone. But a review of these negative reports shows that 30 percent of the patients who developed liver disease were taking both drugs at the same time.

And, Dr. Wolfe notes that liver damage isn't Arava's only problem. There have also been reports of lymphoma, high blood pressure, and a deadly auto-immune disorder associated with the drug.

Find relief for your RA pain AND protect yourself from dangerous side effects

If you have rheumatoid arthritis, and are currently taking or considering taking Arava, be sure to discuss these risks with your doctor. The ACR report recommends that RA patients have tests to measure the level of important liver enzymes called ALT before starting Arava therapy. Once on the drug, patients should have their ALT levels checked each month for the first six months, and if no problems develop, every two to three months afterward. If taking Arava and Rheumatrex together, the ACR calls for assessment of both ALT and another liver enzyme, AST.

But remember that prescription drugs aren't your only option to treat RA. At HSI, we've written about many natural therapies for this debilitating disease. In the July 2001 issue, we told you how mycoplasma microbes can cause RA—and how they can be eradicated by a plant-based antimicrobial agent called Myco+. And in the February 2001 issue, we told you about Wobenzyme, a blend of pancreatic enzymes proven to reduce RA symptoms.

As a proponent of alternative health, I'm all for options. And I know how desperate rheumatoid arthritis patients can be for something, anything, that will relieve their pain. But you deserve to—and need to—know all the risks inherent in each of their alternatives before you make a decision.

To Your Good Health,

Jenny Thompson
Health Sciences Institute

Sources:

- "Arthritis drug may cause liver damage" March 29, 2002 (AP) http://www.intelihealth.com
- "Reports of leflunomide hepatotoxicity in patients with rheumatoid arthritis" American College of Rheumatology http:www.rheumatology.org
- "Arthritis drug should be removed from market" March 28, 2002 http://www.citizen.org

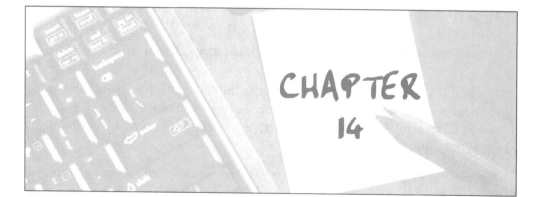

The bandits you trust: Antibiotic laced cows milk

First ran 4/15/2002

It's a little late for April Fool's. And I don't think that Associated Press reporters are known for their senses of humor. But nonetheless, this is the headline that I read on the AP website yesterday:

"Police: Someone is Sneaking onto New York Dairy Farms and Contaminating Milk With Antibiotics."

To borrow a phrase from Dave Barry, I am not making this up. Dairy farmers are actually up in arms that someone has been contaminating their cows and their milk with antibiotics.

I guess they figure that's their job.

Nobody's sneaking—the contamination is blatant

Really, if it's suddenly illegal to contaminate milk, the police are going to have to issue an arrest warrant for nearly every dairy farmer in America. Because every day, most farmers intentionally contaminate their milk—not only with antibiotics, but growth hormones as well.

Most farmers regularly add antibiotics to their animals' feed as a preventative measure, to protect against infections that spread quickly through herds due to the animals' crowded living conditions. (This isn't just true of dairy farmers, it's also widespread practice in raising cattle, chickens, pigs, you name it.) On top of that, dairy cows that are being continuously milked often develop an udder infection called mastitis—and, as a result, are treated with antibiotic injections. (Guess what the leading cause of mastitis in dairy cows is? More on that later.)

The mainstream will tell you that these antibiotics don't make it into the milk supply, and pose no threat to humans. They'll point to the tests that are done on milk before packaging, which are supposed to screen for "contaminants." But many independent tests have shown that the milk on grocery store shelves DOES contain antibiotic residues—either as a result of shoddy screening or the use of illegal antibiotics that can't be detected under current procedures. In fact, in one study conducted by the Center for Science in the Public Interest (CSPI), about 38 percent of milk on grocery store shelves contained antibiotic residues from illegal antibiotics.

You can't discuss antibiotic use in the dairy industry without talking about hormone use as well. Bovine growth hormone use is perhaps an even greater threat—and it is a key cog in this vicious cycle. Recombinant Bovine Growth Hormone (rBGH) is a genetically engineered hormone that is regularly injected into dairy cows to artificially increase their milk production. So how does that relate to antibiotics? Well, cows given rBGH are also MUCH more likely to develop mastitis (even the manufacturer of rBGH warns that it may increase mastitis incidence as much as 80 percent). And you know what mastitis leads to—more antibiotic use, and more antibiotic residues in our milk. (There are other documented risks associated with rBGH, but that's a topic for another time.)

Everyone's red-handed

All of this has been going on for years. And, around the world, groups of concerned consumers have been raising the issue and asking for better controls. For the most part, those concerns have gone unheard.

But now, the police are on the job—because farmers are losing money. (To clarify, it seems they can only sell milk that THEY fill with antibiotics.) Since the incidents began in the fall, about 44,000 gallons of milk have had to be trashed, representing a loss of about $49,000 for the dairy farmers in western New York.

The article says they have "no suspects," although they are looking "any number of places, from animal rights groups opposed to dairy farm practices to disgruntled farmers or employees."

Yes, the dairy farmers just can't seem to imagine who would do something like this—other than themselves, that is.

To Your Good Health,

Jenny Thompson
Health Sciences Institute

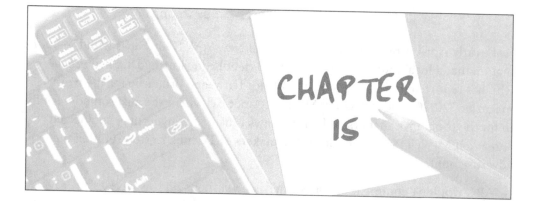

How do you spell relief? Journalist paid to do ad for a major pharma company

First ran 5/2/2002

You may have missed this news story. It didn't get much play in the mainstream press, but it's got everything you want in a good potboiler: corruption, deception, greed, and a pharmaceutical company caught in the spotlight.

On Tuesday, ABC News medical correspondent Dr. Nancy Snyderman was disciplined by the network for making a radio commercial for Tylenol. Her punishment: a suspension of one week, without pay.

There's so much going on here I hardly know where to begin.

Shucks, who knew it was wrong?

In early April, ABC was confronted by the New York Daily News with the information that a local radio station had run a Tylenol ad featuring Dr. Snyderman who has reported on health issues at ABC for ten years, primarily for the newsmagazine "20/20," and for "Good Morning America" where she also sometimes fills in for the program's anchors. When the news broke, Dr. Snyderman apologized and asked McNeil Pharmaceuticals, the makers of Tylenol, to stop running the advertisement.

ABC wouldn't comment on Dr. Snyderman's suspension this week. They say they don't discuss personnel matters. Apparently they don't discuss ethical matters either. But you can bet they were discussing the matters behind closed doors, and they must have been asking the same question that a senior news executive at a rival network asked when he heard the news, "What was she thinking?"

Dr. Snyderman is a seasoned media correspondent who's been recognized with a number of broadcast journalism awards. She's a board-certified surgeon of otolaryngology (ear, nose, and throat) and a trained pediatrician with an established practice in San Francisco. She's been a broadcaster and a doctor for a long time and she certainly knows the rules. What was she thinking? It's transparent. She was thinking she'd get away with it.

Or it's likely that she was just thinking on auto-pilot. Dr. Snyderman had to have known she was stepping across the ethical foul line. But like every physician, she's probably spent so many years rubbing elbows with the drug companies that a little radio plug for Tylenol may have seemed like such a minor lapse that no one would call her on it. And that's confirmed by her punishment. A week off without pay? It's hard to imagine a lighter slap on the wrist. ABC seems to be saying, "Next time, don't get caught."

Medical commentary, bought and sold

Dr. Snyderman got caught this time because she has a high profile and because some hungry reporter at the New York Daily News happened to catch her performance on the radio. But that reporter is probably well aware that this is not an isolated incident. Every newspaper and local TV station in America has a "health" or a "medical" reporter who might enjoy a golf trip, or a consulting job, or a speaking engagement, all arranged and paid for by major pharmaceutical companies. We see this sort of thing happening all the time. And we see the results. When doctors and reporters and high-profile medical correspondents are wined and dined, and golfed and gifted by giant drug corporations, you don't get the urgent research needed to show how natural remedies and supplements can be effective, and you don't get unbiased reporting.

And even though most of us aren't shocked to learn this is happening, we need to stay focused on it and be aware of who's controlling the flow of information from so-called neutral sources. Again, this incident may seem harmless enough but it's just the tip of the iceberg compared to the full scope of corruption and greed going on out there. It's enough to make you reach for a large bottle of acetaminophen.

To Your Good Health,

Jenny Thompson
Health Sciences Institute

Sources:

- New York Daily News
- Executive Speakers Bureau: www.executivespeakers.com

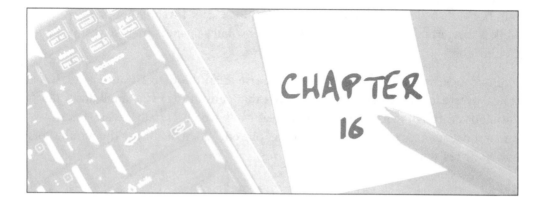

Got antibiotics? Antibiotic use in dairy and livestock farming

First ran 5/8/2002

Last month I told you about a mystery in upstate New York, where someone has been surreptitiously contaminating milk with antibiotics. So far, authorities still don't know who is sabotaging the milk or why. But the situation has focused more attention on the day-to-day contamination that occurs on the vast majority of dairy and cattle farms every day—where farmers routinely force-feed their own animals antibiotics.

Many health authorities and activists have been warning of this danger for years. Yet most people still don't think the threat is real. In fact, we even received a number of disbelieving e-mails in the HSI mailbox after I wrote that first e-Alert. Milk is dangerous? Even contaminated? And by dairy farmers themselves? Couldn't be.

But concerns about farming's role in the rise of antibiotic resistance is not hysterical overreaction. Recent research shows that consuming even small doses of antibiotics through dairy products and meat can have potentially severe, long-range consequences on your health and on our collective health, as the number of antibiotic resistant strains increases.

Doing the math

The use of antibiotics in agriculture is not new. But it seems to be growing each year—and even the mainstream is beginning to take notice. In recent years, a growing body of research has shown that antibiotics are grossly overused in dairy and livestock farming—and that that overuse may play a significant role in the development of human antibiotic resistance.

Consider this: the Union of Concerned Scientists in Cambridge, Mass., found that as much as 80% of the total antibiotic production in the U.S. is used in agriculture—not just on dairy animals, but on every type of livestock and poultry. A substantial portion of that is not even used to fight disease, but to promote growth. Now, a new study out of the University of Maryland supports the idea that agricultural antibiotic use may be introducing new antibiotic-resistant strains of bacteria into the human population—while at the same time making antibiotics less effective in fighting disease.

The study, published in the April 30th issue of the Proceedings of the National Academy of Sciences, evaluated the medical impact of simultaneously using the same antibiotics in livestock animals and as medicine for humans. Using complex mathematical models, the scientists calculated human's every day exposure to animal bacteria and each bacteria's rate of transmission. And based on their research, here's their terrifying conclusion: by the time an antibiotic-resistant bacteria infection could be detected in humans, its course would be irreversible.

I don't mind telling you that the math in this study is way over my head. But even though the model is theoretical, the results are logical—and the science makes a strong argument that something needs to be done.

Who's guarding the henhouse?

Of course, not everyone agrees. One critic of this study is Richard Lobb, a spokesman for the National Chicken Council who dismisses the conclusions as not being "real-world" research. He defends the use of antibiotics by poultry farmers, saying, "They are always used in a responsible manner in the chicken industry."

Hmmm. Why am I not convinced? The National Chicken Council doesn't have anything to gain (or lose) in this issue, do they? The truth is, the mainstream has been dismissing concerns about agricultural antibiotic use for years as baseless and not supported by science. Now, there's more and more science to back it up—but now the research isn't good enough.

The authors of the UM study recommend that authorities regulate and limit the agricultural use of new antibiotics to extend their effectiveness in humans. With all due respect to the Maryland scientists, this isn't a "real-world" solution. We already know that farmers are persistent and can be quite creative in their efforts to sidestep regulations by finding ways to mask their use of antibiotics. As I reported in the first e-Alert on this issue, use of unapproved (and therefore, undetectable) antibiotics in agriculture is widespread. After all, there's a huge economic risk for farmers in NOT using them.

Bringing it all back home

So what can we do? On the large scale, the problem is daunting. But in our own homes, there are steps we can take to protect ourselves and our families. Many people simply choose not to eat animal products. That's one alternative. But if you do eat dairy, eggs, or meats, choose organic whenever possible. Organic farmers do not use antibiotics or growth hormones. One bright spot: organic products are much more accessible that they used to be. You can now find organic dairy and meats—clearly marked—in many mainstream supermarkets.

There's also another way you can help fight the spread of antibiotic-resistant animal bacteria. It's not new advice, but it bears repeating. Cook your meats thoroughly, and be diligent in scrubbing cutting boards and utensils, and always washing your hands well after handling raw meats.

And, remember, farming is a business first and foremost. So given the opportunity to choose whether you want your milk and meat with "antibiotics added" or "guaranteed antibiotic free," speak up—with your wallet. And let the farming industry know that you demand honest information and antibiotic-free foods.

To Your Good Health,

Jenny Thompson
Health Sciences Institute

Sources:

- Proceedings of the National Academy of Sciences 2002;99:6434-6439.

- "Animal Antibiotics Speed Resistance in People" Reuters Health

- "New Alarm Sounded Over Antibiotic Resistance" HealthScoutNews Reporter

A perfect world: Consumer Reports attacks Atkins Diet

First ran 5/9/2002

Last week, Consumer Reports recalled 15,000 glove-compartment organizer kits (a gift sent to new subscribers) because they contained a flashlight that overheated and caused burns. In a press release, Jim Guest, President of Consumer Union, noted that "in a perfect world, the cobbler's children would have the most comfortable shoes, doctors would be the healthiest people," and, I'm paraphrasing here, Consumer Reports would have the basic common sense to test a product before they shipped off 15,000 units.

I'd also add that in a perfect world, magazine editors wouldn't discount medical and diet advice from trained healthcare professionals in favor of their own opinions. But this isn't a perfect world, this is Consumer Reports.

Before I get off on a tangent, let me back up a little bit and tell you what's got me going. Today the mail brought the June issue of Consumer Reports with this cover story: "The Truth about Dieting." Dieting? You've heard me say it before: Consumer Reports should be telling me which dryer won't burn my clothes. Or even which diet powder tastes best or dissolves fastest in water. But not testing and rating which diets THEY deem the healthiest! To be honest I haven't even read the entire article yet. Because once I came across a sidebar titled, "Atkins diet: What's wrong with it?" I was so outraged, I had to sit down and write to you right away.

Send in the "experts"

The "Atkins diet" referred to here is, of course, the popular diet program of Dr. Robert C. Atkins, the author of "Dr. Atkins' New Diet Revolution." I should mention that Agora, HSI's parent company, had published Dr. Atkins' newsletter in the past, so we've had the opportunity to meet and work with this pioneer of complementary medicine, not to mention to read countless media attacks hurled at him (though few have donned headlines as biased and misrepresentative as this one).

The report launches straight into a barrage of the most negative claims, saying the nutrition establishment has denounced Dr. Atkins' diet (I'd be very interested to find out who this "nutrition establishment" is), and an "expert panel of nutritionists" (members, no doubt, of the nutrition establishment) condemned the diet as ineffective and a health hazard. This panel was convened by the American Heart Association, the very same people who once lent their logo to Pop-Tarts, promoting them as a heart-healthy food.

The mini-article then details a study in which overweight volunteers were split into two groups. One group followed the Atkins diet (high protein and fat, but almost zero carbohydrates), and the other group followed what CR calls a "standard" low-fat, low-calorie, high-carbohydrate diet. After 12 weeks, the Atkins group had lost more than twice that of the low-fat group. (It also notes that three times as many people from the "standard group" dropped out altogether.) Yet the article still somehow tap dances around those points and paints the entire program as "unsound."

The leader of the study, Gary Foster, Ph.D., clinical director of the weight-and-eating disorders program at the University of Pennsylvania, is held out by Consumer Reports as the expert. His conclusion: "If I had to say whether the Atkins diet is good or bad, I'd say I still don't know." So why in the world would CR lead off the very same article with such an entirely inappropriate attack, while stopping to genuflect before the AHA expert panel of nutritionists?

Clear results, foggy reporting

If you can get past the propaganda and read the actual information, the statistics clearly support Atkins as the most effective and maintainable diet approach. So shouldn't the headline read, "Atkins diet: Our Test Debunks the Experts"?

And when they trot out a table showing the success rates of 6 diets, where's Dr. Atkins? Missing in action. Jenny Craig is there. Weight Watchers is there. But no Dr. Atkins. Despite the fact that, and I am quoting now, "Of the 10 best-selling diet authors we asked about in our questionnaire, Atkins stood out from the rest. Eighteen percent of all the dieters said they'd read one of his books. That was more than four times as many as had read any of the others. And 34 percent said that his advice helped them to lose weight and keep it off."

So their own readers, the very people upon whose experiences they built this report, had very positive results with this diet. But obviously, someone at Consumer Reports didn't like the those results, so they found a way to bury Dr. A. with omission and negative "expert" rhetoric, forcing you to read very carefully to walk away with any facts.

A reporter in sheep's clothing

I wish Consumer Reports would simply do what they're supposed to do. This cover story on diets is sandwiched between an article on how to choose a PDA (personal digital assistant) and which facial tissue is best. That's exactly what I need from Consumer Reports. And that's all I need.

As many of you know, this isn't the first time I've complained about CR overstepping its bounds. Last August they reported on milk, singing its praises and ignoring a multitude of milk-related health problems. A month later they told us how to manage diabetes. That's exactly what I don't need from Consumer Reports.

But since they had to insert themselves in the world of our health, they owe it to their readers—and, quite frankly, to Dr. Atkins—to conduct a true round of testing and reporting on Dr. Atkins' diet. Had they done that, they would have found plenty of evidence that over the course of more than three decades this diet has helped countless people control diabetes, high blood pressure, and a host of other health problems. They might have pointed out how Dr. Atkins has dedicated his career to combining alternative therapies with conventional medical techniques. And they could have answered the critics who claim that not enough testing has been done on his diet with the information that the Dr. Robert C. Atkins Foundation has awarded a number of unrestricted research grants to, among others, Duke University, the University of Connecticut, and Harvard University, to study controlled carbohydrate research.

So please, Consumer Reports, just be what you are and go back to product testing in your imperfect world. We subscribe for one reason: for you to test and report on air conditioners and microwave ovens, tissues and PDAs. But please keep your reporters' unqualified biases out of our healthcare. And please, don't send us any more flashlights.

To Your Good Health,

Jenny Thompson
Health Sciences Institute

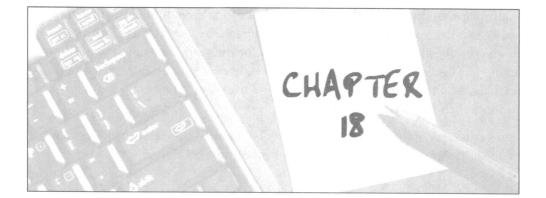

Running scared: Is the FDA's labeling policy in your best interest?

First ran 5/28/2002

Consumption of antioxidant vitamins in the amounts contained in this product may reduce the risk of certain kinds of cancer." If this exact statement were to appear on a dietary supplement label with no disclaimer from the FDA, who would it hurt? Would you and I, health consumers be put at risk as the FDA has insisted time and again? Or, rather, would it be the bottom line of pharmaceutical companies that would be at risk? Sorry, but I sometimes enjoy stating the obvious. But let's be realistic…it's almost impossible to imagine how any of us would suffer a threat to our health from the claim above or from the absence of the FDA disclaimer.

If you're like me, you've got a dozen or more supplements at home that carry a notice that the ingredients have not been evaluated by the FDA. Personally, this disclaimer doesn't affect me in the least. But for the many consumers who come across this disclaimer for the first time, this statement is often interpreted as a warning. And that's exactly how the FDA and the pharmaceutical companies want consumers to feel: warned away.

But the days of the FDA disclaimer may be numbered, side-tracked—finally— by the First Amendment, complements of the Supreme Court.

Winding legal road

Last week the FDA published a notice in the Federal Register, titled "Request for comment on First Amendment Issues." The agency is seeking comments from the public to determine if its product labeling and advertising restrictions are constitutional. (Anyone who cares to weigh in on this topic has until July 30, 2002, to submit comments, and responses to those comments must be received by September 13, 2002.)

In the notice, the agency said, "Recent case law has emphasized the need for not imposing unnecessary restrictions on speech." Which is a coy way of saying that recent case law—the direct result of lawsuits brought against the FDA—has focused on the agency's long-standing policy to restrict freedom of speech.

So far, the decisions of various courts have placed the legal burden on the FDA to prove that claims made by the manufacturers of dietary supplements are false. Throughout the legal process, the FDA has maintained that its primary mission is to protect the public health, which overrides all concerns about First Amendment issues. Fortunately, this argument has not held water in any of the cases, including the case that went before the Supreme Court.

In the most recent ruling in April, the Supreme Court ruled 5 to 4 that the FDA could not block pharmacists from advertising drugs reformulated from bulk supplies. The agency claimed that its ban prevented pharmacists from disseminating false information. A majority of the justices were not swayed, recognizing the language of commercial transaction as "commercial speech," which is entitled to First Amendment protection as long as it's truthful and not misleading.

Who serves public health?

The critical response to the FDA notice has been mixed. Some consumer groups (such as the Center for Science in the Public Interest) believe public health will be harmed if the claims on supplement labels are not regulated. But clearly, the public health is harmed when consumers are driven away from the positive healthy effects of hundreds of supplements that are proven to be effective.

Are there snake oil salesmen out there who would mislead consumers? Of course—there always have been and there always will be. That's why consumers have the responsibility to be diligent about educating themselves when they choose any pharmaceutical or dietary supplement.

Without getting into the constitutionality of the agencies or the benefit of their existence, the simple fact is that the FDA has long overstepped its regulatory bounds by enforcing this misguided disclaimer at all. If anyone is charged with protecting consumers from false claims, it's the Federal Trade Commission. The FDA's mandate is to evaluate the safety and effectiveness of pharmaceuticals, foods, cosmetics, etc. So who does it protect when it takes the unnecessary step of requiring labels to carry this disclaimer? Not the health of the taxpayers. It protects the giant drug companies who stand to lose millions if more and more consumers choose to improve their health with supplements and reduce their need for high priced pharmaceuticals.

Voices of many

So is the FDA now prepared to budge on its long-standing labeling policy—after numerous court challenges and losses? Absolutely not. If the agency is genuinely considering a specific policy change, it wasn't outlined it in the Federal Register notice. Furthermore, this comment was included: "FDA will continue to regulate commercial speech as part of its mandate. In particular, FDA intends to defend the act (Federal Food, Drug, and Cosmetic Act) against any constitutional challenges." To me, that sounds like an agency ready to step up the battle.

Whatever its intentions, there's no doubt that this is a rare opportunity for opinions to be heard. Whether you're a First Amendment scholar or simply a concerned citizen, your comments are important. HSI will be submitting a comment, and I urge you to do so as well.

If you would like to read the entire FDA notice, you can access the Federal Register online at http://www.gpo.gov. From there you'll find a link to the Federal Register. In its notice, the FDA sets forth 9 questions that are not meant to be exhaustive, but rather a jumping off point. They encourage the public to address these and/or other related questions. You can submit comments by going to http://www.fda.gov/dockets/ecomments.

Has the FDA seen the light? They have—and it's not to their liking. Will they give in and give up this self-appointed regulatory power they seized many years ago? Certainly not without a sustained fight. But what matters right now is that all of us have a chance to add our voices and have our say in what might eventually prove to be a turning point in the deregulation of dietary supplements.

To Your Good Health,

Jenny Thompson
Health Sciences Institute

Sources:

- "Request for comment on First Amendment Issues," Federal Register, 5/16/02

- Reuters Health, 5/15/02

- "Challenging FDA Censorship," Reasonline.com

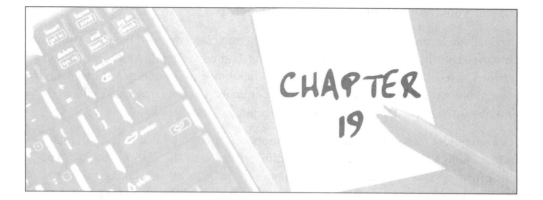

The whistle blower: Physicians on the payroll of the drug companies

First ran 6/6/2002

Greed...corruption...invasions of medical privacy...

Sounds like a chapter out of a John Grisham novel—or a Congressional hearing. But it isn't. It's the latest scandal brought to us by the big drug companies. And it may already have passed through a town near you.

It comes from a New York Times article that delivers plenty of dark drama: drug company greed, unscrupulous sales tactics, corrupt doctors, misuse of a popular FDA-approved drug, a whistle blower, a federal investigation, and even a few "smoking guns."

On the inside

Dateline: Boston 1997. Dr. David P. Franklin contacts a lawyer to file suit against his employer, the pharmaceutical company, Warner-Lambert. Dr. Franklin admits, "I was terrified." Executives at Warner-Lambert had threatened to make him a scapegoat if he went public with his concerns about certain company practices that Dr. Franklin describes as "an illegal marketing scheme that put patients at risk."

Throughout most of the '90s Warner-Lambert (acquired by Pfizer in 2000) manufactured a prescription drug called Neurontin, approved by the FDA for the very specific use of helping to control epileptic seizures for patients already taking another epilepsy drug. But the marketing geniuses at W-L had much bigger plans for Neurontin, which brings us to the first two smoking guns.

In a voice-mail message that's now entered as evidence in Dr. Franklin's lawsuit, a W-L executive told sales reps that in order to market Neurontin effectively they would have to promote it to fight pain, as well as bipolar and other psychiatric uses, in addition to epilepsy. But independent researchers say that Neurontin simply doesn't work for some of those uses and, if used inappropriately, it can cause serious adverse reactions. Dr. Franklin even has internal company documents showing that sales reps encouraged doctors to "experiment" by prescribing Neurontin to treat attention deficit disorder in children. (Yes, you read that right, they are experimenting on our children!)

But the sales reps went much further than simple encouragement. They crossed the line.

Dark shadows

Unfortunately they crossed the line with the help of quite a few doctors who did something completely unprofessional and inexcusable.

In a so-called "shadowing program," W-L paid 75 to 100 doctors for allowing sales reps to sit in during patient exams. This invasion of privacy, condoned by doctors who were trusted by their patients, is truly shocking.

At the conclusion of the exams the sales reps gave "recommendations" on what medicines to prescribe. The doctors were paid $350 or more for each day the sales people were allowed to spend in the exam rooms. Hundreds of patients were affected by this program, but whether or not any of them knew that the person sitting in for their exam was a pharmaceutical salesperson is unclear.

The highest bidders

Can it get any worse? Oh, we're just getting started. Court documents show that doctors who prescribed high volumes of Neurontin were rewarded with additional payments for "consulting" or "speaking" fees. Unfortunately, this sort of practice between doctors and drug companies is not uncommon. For instance, in an unrelated case, a doctor in California allowed a sales rep to attend an exam of a breast cancer patient who was not told at the time that the man was a drug company employee. The doctor was paid $500. (The patient later sued both her doctor and the drug company and the case was settled out of court.)

These sorts of sales tactics have become business as usual for the giant drug companies who spend billions of dollars in their attempts to encourage physicians to prescribe their products. In fact, 37 percent of the doctors who participated in a recent Maryland survey said they had accepted compensation from drug companies in return for prescriptions of their drugs.

Now—want to know how you helped pay for some of those prescriptions? Dr. Franklin's lawsuit has led to a federal investigation claiming that Medicaid paid tens of millions of dollars for Neurontin prescriptions written for untested uses. Those were our tax dollars at work for Warner-Lambert!

Publish or perish

As if all of that weren't enough, Dr. Franklin's case also reveals that Warner-Lambert attempted to influence doctors to prescribe Neurontin by paying them to write medical journal articles that would place Neurontin in a positive light. Offering yet another "smoking gun," W-L internal memos reveal that a marketing firm often wrote the first drafts of articles that were then reviewed by W-L executives before being sent to medical journals for publication.

Court papers show that W-L paid the marketing firm $12,000 to write each article, then paid $1,000 to the doctors who agreed to serve as "authors." This ghost writing, which is an insidious and dishonest form of marketing, is quite common among drug companies.

Old dog, old tricks

So what's going on today with the principals in this drama?

Dr. Franklin—a former research fellow at Harvard Medical School—is currently the director of market research at Boston Scientific, a company that develops medical devices. Reflecting on his time at Warner-Lambert, he says the thing that was most troubling was the pressure they put on him to encourage doctors to prescribe Neurontin in much higher doses than it was approved for. He says, "It was untried ground. I recognized that my actions may be putting people in harm's way."

And Pfizer, through a spokesperson, offers this defense of the ongoing legal mess: "The actions that allegedly occurred took place well before Pfizer completed its merger with Warner-Lambert. It is firm and established Pfizer policy not to allow our sales representatives to make inappropriate claims or encourage off-label use of any of our medicines."

Why am I not convinced? Is this really just an isolated case in an industry that's otherwise honest and has our best interests in mind? The answer to that depends on who you choose to believe: an international drug company spokesperson, or a whistle blower who's seen the dark labyrinth from the inside.

To Your Good Health,

Jenny Thompson
Health Sciences Institute

Sources:

■ "Suit Says Company Promoted Drug in Exam Rooms" New York Times, May 15, 2002

Pretty in pink: Drug companies work the system to extend profitable patents

First ran 6/18/2002

Imagine if we lived in a world where you could get a promotion at work just by changing the color of your shirt. Or you could have more friends simply by using paper bags instead of plastic.

I know, it sounds completely absurd. But for patent drugs, scenarios like these are also surprisingly common.

A new beginning

First some history. As you know, the poor drug companies spend many years and many millions (or billions) of dollars creating a new drug. Then as soon as they get a patent and it hits the market all these upstart generic drug companies come along, and like circling sharks they wait for the patent to expire. As soon as it does, the generics hit market and undercut the price until they start selling more of the product than the former patent holder does. At that point what do the drug giants have to show for all their efforts? Just a few billion dollars in profits and a drug they can no longer call their very own.

But before you start to feel too sorry for them…

There's a nice little loophole they can put to use that extends the life of a drug's patent for two and a half years. And when the drug is a popular, high-profile product, that can mean a very lucrative final run at huge profits before the final bell rings.

Playing dress up

The loophole is simple and effective: claiming that their drug has a new use or a newly added chemical property, the drug company applies for a patent extension. Now that may sound reasonable, but consider this: the patent can even be extended if the only change is a new packaging of the drug. When the extension is granted the reformulated drug has 30 additional months of peak earning power before the generics close in for the kill and bring the price down to earth.

Of course, patents can be extended only if the FDA approves the reformulated drug. But this would appear to be a mere rubber-stamping formality. Just look at the numbers. Between 1989 and 2000, a full two-thirds of all the prescription drugs approved by the FDA were nothing more than modified versions of existing drugs. And some of them weren't even modified—they were identical to drugs already on the market. Meanwhile, only a scant 15 percent of the drugs approved during that period could be considered genuinely "new."

Naming names!

Among the popular reformulated drugs currently on the market there are some brand names I'm sure you'll recognize. The allergy drug Claritin, for instance, was recently reformulated to become Clarinex. Prilosec, an ulcer medication, became Nexium. And—this is my favorite—Sarafem, prescribed for relief of premenstrual irritability, is a pink and lavender capsule that is otherwise identical to one of the true celebrities of prescription drugs: Prozac. Prozac! So they made the pill prettier and got a new slogan, forcing users to pay patent prices for two and a half more years. Plus, I wonder how these irritable women would react if they had any idea they were actually being given Prozac.

All of this information comes from a new research report released last month by the National Institute for Health Care Management (NIHCM) Foundation, a non-profit organization that promotes improvements in health care access, management and quality.

The report also found that the so-called "new" drugs with modified formulas were priced much higher than the drugs they replaced. In other words, the drug giants take their star performers, dress them up in their Sunday best, and then jack up the prices—all with the formal blessing of our friends at the FDA.

Keeping it real

There's currently a bill pending in Congress (Greater Access to Affordable Pharmaceuticals Act) that would close these patent loopholes and give our pocketbooks a little relief. But if history is any judge, don't expect the pharmaceutical companies to come out the losers.

I would add to that; if you must rely on a prescription drug, ask your doctor about the specific history of that drug. Otherwise you might get Prozac, renamed and dressed up in a colorful new and more expensive package.

...and another thing

As I mentioned last week, we continue to receive e-mails and postings on the forum in response to the e-Alert I sent you about the debate over smallpox vaccine ("A shot in the arm; a shot in the dark" 6/10/02). A reader named MBJ wrote with a point of view shared by several others:

"It seems that the good of the many may jeopardize a FEW but, isn't that what it is all about? We have to think about what will help the most people. As a nurse I think, generally, that we have to protect the masses. Yes, some will perish. I'm just not convinced that we should spread panic when it seems that vaccination may save thousands of lives if available."

I agree, MBJ, that we should not spread panic. But we do need to carefully look at all sides of this matter, even if it means we have to look at some frightening things. If someone were giving us overwhelming evidence that we were on the verge of an outbreak of smallpox, measures to protect millions at the peril of a few would be in our combined best interest. But right now the threat of smallpox being introduced into the population is only a possibility. And forcing vaccinations, or any medical decisions, to deal with a possibility could very well hurt more people than it would protect.

But the larger question here is: how much personal freedom and how many civil liberties should we risk to protect ourselves against something that might happen? I don't believe there are any easy answers, but I'm certain that we can expect the debate to intensify in the upcoming months.

To Your Good Health,

Jenny Thompson
Health Sciences Institute

Sources:

- "Changing Patterns of Pharmaceutical Innovation" May, 2002 Research Report, National Institute for Health Care Management
- "Majority of New Medicines Approved in the 1990s Were Altered Versions of Older Drugs" Press Release, National Institute for Health Care Management
- "New Medicines Seldom Contain Anything New, Researchers Find" International Herald Tribune

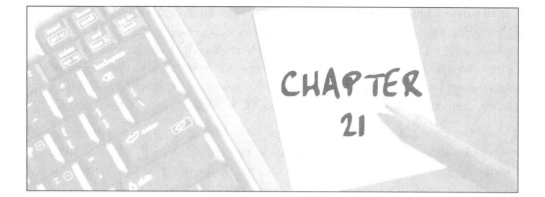

Fore!
Top medical journal
eases ethics policy

First ran 6/20/2002

There was a seismic shift in medical journalism last week, and the Chicago Tribune headline said it all: "Top Medical Journal Eases Ethics Policy."

For those of us who look to the journals for reliable medical reporting, this is not good news. But there really isn't much we can do about it at this point other than marvel at the absurd statements that are being offered to defend this astounding lapse of judgment.

Standards going South

The "top medical journal" in question is the New England Journal of Medicine, once a paragon of virtue with the strictest conflict-of-interest standards among medical research publications. But all of that went South when editor Jeffrey M. Drazen and executive editor Gregory D. Curfman co-signed an editorial that conceded defeat to the blizzard of drug company bucks. They certainly tried to put a good face on it, which brings us to Absurd Statement #1: "With these modifications in policy, we can prevent financial interests from infringing on the editorial content of the Journal."

Nice try, guys! But what's really happening here is the exact opposite: financial interests have deeply infringed on the editorial content of the NEJM. Drazen and Curfman are trying to make it sound like they're fighting the good fight when they're actually lying down and throwing in the towel.

The fact is, the Journal is completely reversing the rules regarding conflict-of-interest for authors of review articles and editorials. The old NEJM policy stated that authors may not have ANY financial interest in a company (or its competitor) discussed in an article. That seems reasonable. After all, if Doctor Smith is singing the praises of Brand X, and if the makers of Brand X have written Doc Smith a fat check, you would have to consider his "expert" opinion to be little more than a paid advertisement.

The new policy adds just one word. But what a big word it turns out to be. Between "any" and "financial" now insert "significant." And what's the going rate of "any significant financial interest?" Any amount of gifts or money that exceeds $10,000. So, for instance, a set of the finest golf clubs, two first class airline tickets to Palm Springs, a week in an Executive Suite of a four-star hotel, and a couple thousand dollars in spending money for meals and greens fees would not be considered significant.

Did someone change the definition of "significant" when I wasn't looking?

Payday for influence

For a moment, let's pretend we were born yesterday and ask, "Why would they do this?" Which brings us to Absurd Statement #2: Editor Drazen claims that without this policy change NEJM won't be able to find any experts to contribute reviews or editorials who have not accepted money or gifts from pharmaceutical companies because "there are not enough of them around."

So what Drazen would have us believe is that nearly every doctor and researcher who is qualified to offer an expert opinion has accepted gifts, stipends or cold cash from major drug companies—but not more than $10,000. More amazing is that he would also have us believe that $9,999 would not influence an author to bias an article to benefit his benefactor.

Is anyone buying ANY of this?

At least one person is: Dr. Catherine DeAngelis, editor of the Journal of the American Medical Association, who gives us Absurd Statement #3: "I really think this is much ado about nothing. The New England Journal joined the rest of us by adding the word, 'significant.' That's all that's new."

Put another way, anyone who is surprised by this is, supposedly, naive. DeAngelis and Drazen are saying they've seen the flood of drug money pouring over the dam and can't do a thing about it. Then they try to shrug it off as if they're innocent bystanders with no power and no responsibility.

Spineless leadership

I really don't know which situation is worse here: the editors who are willing to compromise the integrity of their once venerable journals, or the belief that drug money has stuffed the pockets of just about every qualified author.

Looking ahead, it's easy to see the clear message that this relaxed journalistic integrity will send to young medical authors just starting out: it's fine to accept some money, even a lot of money, but just don't exceed the "significant" limit. I'll let Dr. DeAngelis have the final Absurd Statement—#4: "What matters is the quality of their opinions. Is the article balanced? Is it fair? Is it true? Bias has a distinct odor, and it's up to us to smell it before publication."

And after publication, what's that distinct odor that lingers? Drug company money. Lots of it. And plenty more where that came from.

...and another thing

Well, as Tom Brokaw and the rest of the country continue the smallpox debate, so do we.

Margaret D. wrote to ask about how the vaccine itself can transmit a virus (see "...and another thing" in yesterday's e-Alert for the answer to that question). She also agreed that "the government could and will force vaccinations in the case of biological warfare," but then goes on to quote a friend of hers, a "Ph.D. clinician," who says, "to think the government can force someone to take a vaccination is ludicrous. If that were true, we wouldn't have the problem today with getting all kids to be immunized."

Unfortunately, Margaret, you're right and your friend is wrong. It does sound ludicrous—and I wish it were—but the fact is that provisions are being made for the most extreme responses to a smallpox outbreak, and forced vaccination is one of them. The Center for Law and the Public's Health at Georgetown and Johns Hopkins Universities has prepared a "Model State Emergency Health Powers Act" that would give public health officials the power to use state militia to enforce vaccination during declared health emergencies.

This of course is a much different situation than that of immunizing school-age kids for various diseases. School principals still don't have the authority to call out the National Guard to force mumps and measles vaccinations...yet.

To Your Good Health,

Jenny Thompson
Health Sciences Institute

Sources:

- "Financial Associations of Authors"
- The New England Journal of Medicine, 346:1901-1902
- "New England Journal Loosens Rules on Authors' Ties to Firms" The Wall Street Journal
- "Top Medical Journal Eases Ethics Policy" The Chicago Tribune

CHAPTER
22

Barbarians at the garden gate: Will voluntary guidelines between docs and drug companies be effective?

First ran 6/27/2002

Can you feel it? Can you sense the electricity in the air? That's the exciting buzz of change on the way. Because come next Monday, everything will be different.

As of next Monday, July 1, 2002, pharmaceutical companies and their salespeople will have new guidelines to follow concerning their relationships with physicians. These guidelines are clear and detailed. But above all, they are…voluntary.

First the facts…

Last April, the Executive Committee of the Pharmaceutical Research and

Manufacturers of America (PhRMA) unanimously adopted a new marketing code that will, to use its phrase, "govern the pharmaceutical industry's relationships with physicians." This is in response to a rising tide of criticism about drug company perks offered to doctors. The perks can range from the low rent, such as filling up a doctor's car with gas, to far more luxurious all-expense paid junkets to conferences.

PhRMA would have us believe that these new rules of the road will rein in the sometimes wild excesses drug salesmen use to win over doctors and healthcare professionals. But PhRMA is not a governing body. It's a trade organization. And one of its primary functions is to polish the public image of its industry and its membership that includes giant drug companies such as Bristol-Myers Squibb, Pfizer, Novartis, Merck, etc.

So, does the new code have teeth? In a word: no.

First of all, let me repeat: it's voluntary. They're asking salespeople to show restraint even if their competition does not. A long shot proposition at best.

Second: for more than a decade the AMA has had very similar guidelines in place. In fact, they revised them last summer and then kicked off a high-profile campaign to get the word out to doctors and pharmaceutical reps. If those guidelines didn't have any effect, who is really going to pay any attention to this new "code"?

And third: fortunately for the sales reps, these clear and detailed guidelines are full of hazy language and loopholes. For instance, throughout the document you'll find phrases like "reasonably necessary," and "appropriate use," and "reasonable compensation"—all providing plenty of "reasonable and appropriate" wiggle room when it comes to interpretation. And the code still allows the irresistible "consultant" loophole—that is: drug companies can hire doctors as "consultants" and send them to conferences, all expenses paid.

Can't we all just get along?

Okay, I'll try to play nice for a minute.

The PhRMA code is not a set of binding regulations. It's a set of guidelines. And that's a good thing. In general, we work with our peers to find a consensus of values and boundaries. Then, if everyone isn't on the same page, well at least we have a page that we can point to and say, "there, that's our ideal," and we hope everyone will strive to meet the standards of that ideal.

But down in the trenches it's a different story. The salesman is motivated to sell in a marketplace where the competition is fierce. So it would seem that if anyone is going to enforce this code it would have to be the only ones who are present at the point of contact with the pharmaceutical reps: the doctors. If the doctors "just say no," then the problem vanishes. But so far, there haven't been a lot of "no's." (Want proof? Remember when I told you that the New England Journal of Medicine announced it had to change it's editorial policy because there weren't enough doctor/authors who were not receiving compensation from the pharmaceutical companies?)

Who's the loser? You and me, of course. The ones, for instance, who pay a premium price for a patent medicine when the doctor could just as easily write a generic prescription; the ones who pay more than we need to because a doctor over-prescribes a medication; or the patients who could be effectively treated with an inexpensive supplement but are prescribed a drug instead.

Back to the garden

I'm reminded of a story I once heard about a boy who saw his father put a small padlock on a garden shed. He said, "Dad, that little padlock wouldn't keep anyone out." And his father said, "I know. It's just there to keep the honest honest."

At best, that's what the PhRMA code is: a flimsy padlock.

...and another thing

Earlier this week I told you about a compound found in broccoli and broccoli sprouts that may lead to advances in fighting peptic ulcers and stomach cancer. The next day I heard from HSI member Howard F. who had this to say:

"Don't you keep up? Sprouts are bad, not good. Bacteria from the growing medium."

Howard is right—to an extent. In recent years there have been reported cases of people getting sick from bacteria growing in sprouts. These are isolated cases, however, and the reaction from sprout growers has been a marked increase in quality control. But to be on the safe side it wouldn't hurt to ask the manager of your local health food store about what measures are taken to insure that their sprouts are safe. If you still feel uncertain about the bacteria question, then you can avoid eating the sprouts raw. Cooking sprouts in a stir-fry dish, for instance, should kill off any bacteria that may be lingering. Or you can likely find sprouts in supplement form at your health food store or online.

To Your Good Health,

Jenny Thompson
Health Sciences Institute

Sources:

- "PhRMA Code on Interactions with Healthcare Professionals" Pharmaceutical Research and Manufacturers of America
- "PhRMA Adopts New Marketing Code" Press release, Pharmaceutical Research and Manufacturers of America
- "Drug Industry Adopts Guidelines on Giveaways to Doctors" The Washington Post
- "Drug-marketing Perks Curbed" The Washington Times

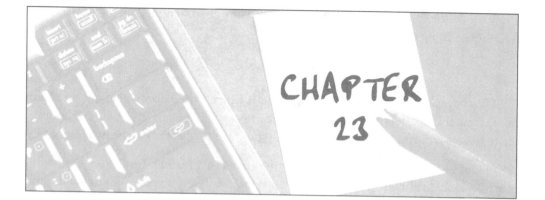

Glory days: Viagra and major league baseball

First ran 7/8/2002

Today: a baseball story for the dog days.

We begin with a team mired in the cellar of the National League East—the Philadelphia Phillies. Even though they have two infielders good enough to be starters in the upcoming All Star Game, their pitching is inconsistent, their hitting untimely, and their fielding abysmal. On July 19, 20 and 21 they will host a series with the team that holds first place in their division, the Atlanta Braves. The Braves are excellent players in every respect, and their won/lost record is currently the best in baseball.

What do the Phillies need? Isn't it obvious? They need Viagra. And, believe it or not, they're going to get it.

Just a little over the top

If you haven't heard the news, Viagra is (this is where Dave Barry would say "and I am not making this up") an official sponsor of Major League Baseball (MLB). Which leads me to believe it must be the official erectile dysfunction medication of the two leagues.

You may have seen the television advertisements that feature Texas Ranger first baseman Rafael Palmeiro as the most recent Viagra Guy. And you've got to hand it to him—he does a pretty good job of keeping a straight face.

What you may not be aware of is the unusual promotional campaign cooked up by Viagra and Major League Baseball. Four National League teams (the Braves, Marlins, Mets and Phillies), and three American League teams (Angels, A's and Rangers), will each host a special series of games in their home ballparks this summer to honor a winning era of their respective franchise. Viagra will be the highly visible sponsor of all of these series for which the official title is—again, no kidding—"The Triumphant Glory Series."

That's right: Triumphant Glory, brought to you by Viagra.

Mommy, what's Viagra?

Viagra and Major League Baseball certainly have every right to buy and sell advertising as they please, but is it really appropriate to peddle Viagra at family oriented events where a large number of children will be present? And if you think I'm talking about the sexual connotation, I'm not—even though it's going to be an interesting challenge for mommy to explain to the kids what Viagra is.

Two things are being sold here. Viagra is selling a message that equates their product with victory, championships and Triumphant Glory (and I'm not going to touch that one with a ten-foot pole—pardon the expression). And Pfizer, the maker of Viagra, is quietly selling this sub-text message: drugs are just as wholesome as baseball, they solve problems, and they're good for us. This message—sent over and over and over again on television, on the radio, in magazines, and now at the ballpark—is helping to create a culture that's becoming dependent on prescription drugs. And dependency is a good thing—when you're the one making billions of dollars a year selling it.

And keep this in mind: Most baseball promotional dates are aimed at kids. In Philadelphia, for instance, other promotional giveaways this season include a growth chart, a kid's lunch box, a bobble head doll of the Phillie Phanatic, and a Spongebob Squarepants rally towel. Fans who attend the Triumphant Glory Series will receive a painter's cap printed with the Viagra logo, and I'm sure that when the school year begins, many of those caps are going to show up at grade schools in Philadelphia, Atlanta, Oakland and other cities. Is this is a small thing? Sure. It's subtle. It's practically subliminal. And that's the most effective way to get the "feel good" message through.

Is that a Valium in your pocket?

According to the New England Journal of Medicine, the money spent on direct-to-consumer advertising for prescription drugs tripled between 1996 and 2000, when the pharmaceutical industry spent $2.5 billion on advertising. Without a doubt, this year it will be considerably more. And much like the giant tobacco companies, one of their primary target audiences is the impressionable minds of kids—the future drug buyers of America.

Right now Claritin is the only other patent drug that's an official MLB sponsor. But with Viagra popping up in ballparks (sorry, I couldn't resist), can Ritalin bat day, or Prozac backpack night, or Valium thermos twilight doubleheader be far behind?

...and another thing

An HSI member named Paul has posted a message in the HSI Forum under the heading "Carotid Arteries." Paul's message is a response to a recent e-Alert ("Therapy of the Gods" 6/26/02) in which another member, Fred V., mentioned that he has carotid arteries. Here's Paul's comment:

"Why not tell him about EDTA chelation treatments? It will clear all blockages from the cardiovascular system without risk or side affects. I speak from experience."

Paul's comment was quickly followed by this very informative message from TS, an M.D. who has some strong opinions about chelation:

"I'm responding to the statement that chelation will 'clear all blockages from the cardiovascular system'. It won't, and don't get chelation if that's what you're expecting to accomplish. Don't get me wrong—I'm a BIG supporter of chelation, and am not real fond of carotid surgeries. It's a dangerous, expensive, over-performed procedure, but pays a lot of surgeons' bills.

"Although chelation won't actually open up a carotid blockage significantly—it's a big, fat artery—it will improve function in the tiny arteries that are supplying the brain (and other organs)—and those are the ones that are really important. If we have an artery that's 90% (or more) blocked, then our bodies have already developed a collateral system to supply that organ, otherwise that organ would be pretty much dead already.

"Chelation helps protect and optimize this alternate circulation. So if you do get chelated, don't think you can go back to eating crap and doing the same things that caused your arteries to plug up in the first place, or your collateral arteries will fill up with gunk, too. Chelation is a great therapy, and can often give you a second chance, but it won't let you 'start from scratch.' Your primary circulation is pretty much trashed, and will stay that way. Take care of your new one."

Thanks, Doc, for that thorough and candid opinion. Anyone else have experience or insights into chelation therapy? If so, please drop by the HSI Forum and let us know about it. The more voices, the better.

To Your Good Health,

Jenny Thompson
Health Sciences Institute

Sources:

- Web sites for the Philadelphia Phillies and Major League Baseball "Promotion of Prescription Drugs to Consumers"
- New England Journal of Medicine, 346 #7 "Direct-to-Consumer Prescription Drug Advertising" Kaiser Network AdWatch

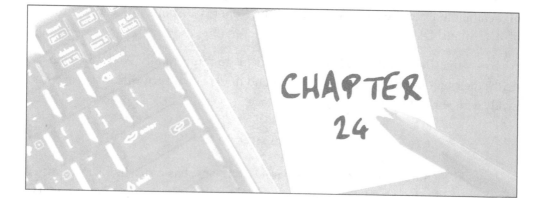

Taking a Brody: New York Times journalist takes on Atkins Diet

First ran 7/10/2002

This past weekend at Wimbledon, Venus and Serena Williams dominated. They each advanced to the final round of the singles championship (little sister Serena won it this year), and then teamed up the next day to win the doubles title—once again.

I watched their doubles match as I browsed through the Sunday New York Times. The cover story in the magazine was a new chapter in another intense volley that's been going on for years in the diet world.

This volley is Brody vs. Atkins. That is: Jane E. Brody, the columnist who writes on health issues for the New York Times, and Robert C. Atkins, M.D., the author of "Dr. Atkins' Diet Revolution."

To say that these two have been adversarial is to put it mildly. And now, suddenly, their face-off has taken a surprising and unexpected turn that may leave Ms. Brody with some high-protein egg on her face.

That was then

I should mention that Agora, HSI's parent company, has published Dr. Atkins' newsletter in the past, so I've met and worked with this pioneer of complementary medicine. Over the course of 30 years, Dr. Atkins has not wavered from his controversial dietary ideas. In a nutshell, Dr. Atkins advises us to eat as much meat and other high protein and high fat foods as we care to, while avoiding starches and refined carbohydrates such as breads, pasta, rice and sugars. This plan has won many millions of readers, but has drawn numerous, often passionate attacks from the nutrition and diet establishment.

Enter Jane E. Brody who has ridiculed the Atkins plan a number of times through the years. In 1999 she wrote a column for the New York Times, in which she scoffed at the diet and gleefully quoted two nutritionists who said, "The Atkins diet is potentially so dangerous that the Surgeon General should probably put a warning on every book Dr. Robert Atkins sells." Finally she dismissively pointed out that no researchers had taken the "Atkins scheme" seriously (although she personally knew four people who tried the diet and had problems with it—apparently that was all the "research" she needed to form a conclusion).

But that was then and this is now. And now Ms. Brody has the opportunity to enjoy a meal of high-fat crow, made possible, ironically, by the very newspaper she writes for.

Low-fat chickens come home to roost

The title of the cover story of the Sunday New York Times Magazine (7/7/02) asks this question: "What if It's All Been a Big Fat Lie?" The article's author, Gary

Taubes, states that "a small but growing minority of establishment researchers have come to take seriously what the low-carb-diet doctors have been saying all along."

Notable among these researchers is Walter Willett, chairman of the department of nutrition at the Harvard School of Public Health. Willett, who is the spokesman for a long-running study that includes data on almost 300,000 subjects, says that the low-fat-is-good-health message is clearly contradicted by their findings. Furthermore, it appears that the extreme focus on the adverse effects of fat may have contributed to the huge upswing of obesity in America.

In the 30+ years that the idea of the low-fat diet has become gospel, the number of obese Americans has been steadily rising, to the point that obesity is now being called an epidemic. Meanwhile, the current NY Times article points out that the Atkins diet may successfully address obesity by controlling blood sugar levels and reducing the intake of empty calories.

Tables turned

In a letter published in the New York Times in 1999, Dr. Atkins responded to the accusations of Ms. Brody, saying, "As a practicing cardiologist, my work is based on helping patients. What motivates Ms. Brody's hostility? She does a disservice to millions who lead healthier lives on my program and to many more who continue to embrace unproductive dietary programs thanks to misinformation of the sort propagated by Ms. Brody."

Perhaps this past Sunday's New York Times article has signaled an important change in direction, moving the conventional wisdom toward the close of an era of unproductive dietary programs and misinformation. Ms. Brody stated correctly in 1999 that there was as yet no major research available to support Dr. Atkins' claims. I'm really looking forward to see how (or if) she'll respond now that her own newspaper has delivered the news that research results have started coming in—and she was wrong.

In 1886 a young newsboy named Steve Brodie jumped off the Brooklyn Bridge and survived. For many years after, a leap from the great bridge was referred to as "taking a Brodie." Maybe the term will be revived and the spelling updated and in 2002 "taking a Brody" will refer to the embarrassment of publicly ridiculing someone that later turns out to be right.

To Your Good Health,

Jenny Thompson
Health Sciences Institute

Sources:

- "What if It's All Been a Big Fat Lie?" Gary Taubes, New York Times Magazine, 7/7/02
- "Weight Loss Report: Personal Health; Doubts Fail to Deter 'The Diet Revolution'" Jane E. Brody, New York Times, May 25, 1999
- "Dr. Atkins Responds" Dr. Robert C. Atkins, Letter, New York Times, June 1, 1999

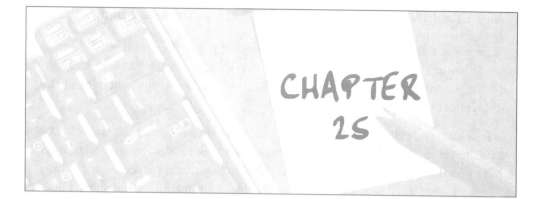

CHAPTER
25

Flying under the radar: Pharmaceutical companies manufacturing own placebo pills

First ran 7/25/2002

Placebo. As a pharmaceutical research tool it's dismissed as nothing but a sugar pill. What could be more innocuous or benign? Even the sound of the word is comforting somehow. In fact, it comes from the Latin word meaning "I shall please." Everything about the word is guileless.

Or so I thought. If you're like me, you'll be shocked—actually more like flabbergasted—to find out that drug research trials bring a whole new meaning to the old Latin idea of "I shall please."

Take two SweetTarts and call me in the morning

There was a time long ago when doctors would prescribe phony medication—sugar pills—to their patients who they regarded as hypochondriacs. They called the pills "placebo" and when the patients reported positive results the idea of the placebo effect was born.

These days, placebo pills are used in clinical trials to measure the true effect of a drug or supplement. They are thought to be made of inert substances designed to have no effect. That's the idea, anyway. But consider this: there's no such thing really as an inert substance. For instance, placebo pills are still called sugar pills. Is sugar inert? Far from it, of course. If you take a sugar pill, your body will have a reaction, especially if you happen to have an insulin disorder. But if you're given that same pill as part of a drug research trial, your reaction becomes a factor in the research.

That may seem like nothing (what real difference could a little boost of sugar make?) but sugar and other supposedly inactive ingredients are not the problem. Not in the least.

Not exactly what we thought it was

When a pharmaceutical company tests its products, where do you suppose they get placebo pills? Do they place an order with a placebo pill manufacturer? Or does Nestle's candy company run a little side business to supply researchers with sugar pills?

Would it surprise you to learn that drug companies make their own placebo pills for research purposes? And that THEY choose the ingredients? And sometimes they purposely put ingredients into the placebos that match those in the drug and will affect the outcome of the trial. And they are not required to disclose the ingredients they use.

Does that sound "inert" or "inactive" to you? Suddenly the idea of a "sugar pill" doesn't seem so innocent anymore.

Before conducting human trials for drugs, pharmaceutical companies are often fully aware of many of the side effects of the products they're testing. So, for instance, if a drug is known to cause dizziness and hypertension, the drug company running the test wants the placebo to have the same side effects. And they have an explanation for this. They say the placebo should mimic the drug being tested so that the control group of the experiment will have side effects similar to the placebo group. Without that, they claim, the results of a blind study would be compromised.

There are plenty of gray areas to debate in that logic, but for the moment let's focus on the idea of what they call an "active placebo," designed to mimic the side effects of a tested drug. And with that in mind let's look at an advertising campaign for the allergy medication called Claritin. In all their TV spots, when it comes to the moment to list the side effects, the voice-over says, "The most common side effects with Claritin, including headache, drowsiness, fatigue and dry mouth, occurred about as often as they did with a sugar pill."

A sugar pill? Really? Just what kind of "sugar pill" were they using that caused headache, drowsiness, fatigue and dry mouth? Sounds to me like a sugar pill with a little something added. But they want us to believe that their powerful medication will produce side effects no more serious than what you'd get with a little dab of sugar.

The cat is still in the bag

I have to thank HSI Panelist Dr. Allan Spreen, MD, who first tipped me off about the little-known world of placebos. Since then, we've also spoken with Dr. Beatrice Golomb, MD, PhD, an assistant professor of medicine at the University of California, San Diego, who has been actively fighting the research establishment's claim that placebos are inactive substances. Dr. Golomb wants scientists to provide a list of placebo ingredients so trial results can be properly evaluated.

To level the playing field, Dr. Golomb suggests that drug companies start divulging all placebo ingredients. She also recommends that a standardized set of placebos be developed that would have known and predictable side effects. This would go a long way toward eliminating the pharmaceutical industry's cynical manipulation of test data.

As you might suspect, the drug companies are not very receptive to her idea of letting go of this aspect of product testing that they have full control over.

Meanwhile, what about physicians and researchers who work independently from the pharmaceutical giants—do they know the truth about placebos supplied by drug companies? Right now it's hard to tell just how widespread this knowledge is. According to the National Center for Complementary and Alternative Medicine at the National Institutes of Health (NIH), the placebo effect is defined as "desirable physiological or psychological effects attributable to the use of inert medications." From that statement it would appear that the NIH either believes that placebos are genuinely inactive, or they're not saying.

Or maybe they're just feeling drowsy, dizzy, irritable and nauseous from a sugar pill someone gave them.

...and another thing

Health care information on the Internet: now there's a subject that gets my attention.

Harris Interactive, a market research company, recently conducted an international survey of Internet users who seek health information. In the four countries surveyed—the U.S., France, Germany and Japan—they found that people who use the Internet as a source to research health concerns think that the information they receive is trustworthy, of good quality and easy to understand.

That's the good news.

The news that I found troubling is that the majority of users in three of those countries (the U.S., France and Japan) believe that the government should regulate health content on the Internet.

I spend quite a bit of time reviewing health related web sites, so I know there's a good deal of information out there that's suspect. But the idea of the government regulating the Internet information I have access to is like saying the government should regulate what books ought to be available to me. I think it's my right to have access to all information and all books, good or bad, because I trust myself to make informed choices on my own without the benefit of government intervention.

I also find it hard to fathom why people who think something is trustworthy, of good quality and easy to understand would want to see it regulated. Do they really imagine that the guidance of a slow-moving bureaucracy would improve the quality and make it even more trustworthy? (Or, more likely, was it how the question was asked...)

Meanwhile, as long as I've got my knives out, I also have a bone to pick with the folks at Harris Interactive who have coined a special phrase to describe those of us who look for health information on the Internet: cyberchondriacs. It's catchy, it's cute, but it's very condescending. And because it draws from the word "hypochondriac," it also implies that we're just slightly off our rockers.

We're not "chondriacs" of any kind—hypo or cyber. We're Internet users who care about our health, both as individuals and as a community. And we certainly don't need the government to "protect us" by deciding what information is good for us.

To Your Good Health,

Jenny Thompson
Health Sciences Institute

Sources:

- "Health Info on Web Should be Regulated, Users Say" Reuters Health, 6/13/02

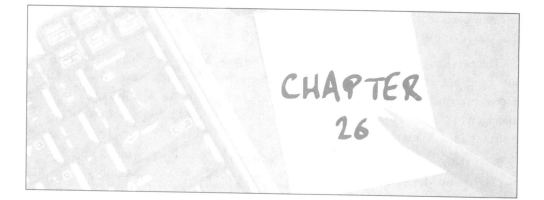

CHAPTER
26

In the trenches with the superbugs: Drug resistant bacteria and overuse of antibiotics

First ran 8/6/2002

They're called "superbugs"—bacteria so determined to survive that they adapt to whatever antibiotics we invent to fight them. This frightening scenario has turned into a dangerous, ongoing battle, just as we at HSI first predicted it would 6 years ago.

With all the frightening upheavals going on in the world right now it's easy to overlook the war being waged on a microscopic level inside our own bodies. But as daunting as it is, the good news is that there are some essential and easy steps you can take to protect yourself and your family.

Michigan battle ground

But first, the bad news. Two weeks ago, doctors in Michigan reported the first case of a new bacterium that is completely resistant to vancomycin—a powerful antibiotic that's so effective that it's referred to as a "last line of defense."

The new drug-resistant bacterium is a variation on Staphylococcus aureus (SA), a superbug that sometimes causes infections in wounds following surgery. SA is the first bacterium considered to be completely resistant to vancomycin. The Michigan doctors managed to catch the infection early and contain it, but they believe that vancomycin-resistant SA will emerge again.

Fred Tenover of the U.S. Centers for Disease Control led the bacterial analysis in Michigan, and said that he and his colleagues fully expect to see more mutated organisms like SA. For several years scientists have been developing new antibiotics called linezolid and quinupristin/dalfopristin to address new mutations of vancomycin-resistant SA. But new strains of SA have already been identified that are resistant to the new drugs.

How does SA find a way to overcome the new drugs so quickly? Gary French, a clinical microbiologist of Guy's & St. Thomas' Hospital in London believes that the problem lies with doctors who are not aware of the risks of over-prescribing antibiotics. French says, "It's extremely worrying."

My feelings exactly. Unfortunately, the dilemma of physicians who are uninformed is just one part of a large problem that begins down on the farm.

Quick fix side effects

In an e-Alert I sent you last May ("Got Antibiotics?" 5/8/02) I told you about the deplorable situation on dairy and cattle farms where farmers routinely force-feed antibiotics to their livestock to prevent disease.

In recent years, a growing body of research has shown that antibiotics are grossly overused in dairy and livestock farming—and that overuse may play a significant role in the development of human antibiotic resistance.

Think the fear of antibiotics in livestock is inflated? Then consider this: as much as 80% of the total antibiotic production in the U.S. is used in agriculture. I don't know about you, but I find that truly shocking. And it's not used on just dairy animals, but on every type of livestock and poultry. What's worse, a substantial portion of it is not even used to fight disease, but to promote growth.

A University of Maryland study released last spring supported the conclusion that agricultural antibiotic use may be introducing new antibiotic-resistant strains of bacteria into the human population. But Richard Lobb doesn't agree. Mr. Lobb is a spokesman for the National Chicken Council and dismisses the conclusions of the Maryland study. He defends the use of antibiotics by poultry farmers, saying, "They are always used in a responsible manner in the chicken industry."

For some reason I don't feel reassured.

Your personal homeland security

Here's a sobering thought: Bacteria can "teach" one another to resist antibiotics.

Bacteria are highly adaptive. When one develops resistance to an antibiotic, it can pass that resistance to similar and even unrelated strains. They do this by passing plasmids, which are DNA-containing organisms, from one to another. Some researchers have suggested this is the reason some microbes that once caused diseases only in animals are now also infecting and killing humans.

The authors of the Maryland study concluded with a recommendation that authorities regulate and limit the agricultural use of new antibiotics. Unfortunately this isn't a "real-world" solution. We've already seen evidence that many farmers can be quite creative in their efforts to sidestep regulations and mask their use of antibiotics.

So what can you do in your own home to protect yourself and your family? If your diet includes dairy, eggs, or meats, choose organic whenever possible. Organic farmers do not use antibiotics or growth hormones, and you can now find organic dairy and meats—clearly marked—in many mainstream supermarkets. It's also important to cook meats thoroughly and be diligent in scrubbing cutting boards and utensils.

And of course, anything you can do to boost your immune system gives your body a much better chance of fighting all bacteria. In other words, eat your vegetables! Cauliflower, cabbage, Brussels sprouts and broccoli have all been shown to have a natural detoxifying effect on your body.

At HSI we regard this growing epidemic of superbugs as one of our primary concerns. As we bring you further reports about resistant bacteria and new antibiotics, I'll also be watching for more information on innovative and natural ways to fight the good fight on the microscopic level.

...and another thing

An HSI member named J.H. recently posted an item on the HSI Forum, asking other members for advice with this question:

"I have a friend recently diagnosed with NASH disease which affects the liver and can lead to other complications. Are there any supplements or alternative therapies anyone has heard about? "

NASH disease—or "non-alcoholic steatohepatitis"—is a condition in which an excessive amount of fat accumulates in the liver. The first half of its name, "non-alcoholic," addresses the fact that the disease is indistinguishable from alcoholic hepatitis. NASH disease is a poorly understood condition that occurs primarily in women, especially those who have diabetes or are overweight. The fat content of the liver can usually be quickly reduced with weight reduction. But there are other methods of addressing the problem, and for those I'll turn to a couple of Forum responses to J.H.'s question.

Olive writes, "Thysillin has long been known as an herbal support for the liver. We have utilized Natures Way 2x standardized extract. Should be available at your health food store." And to that, Leppert adds, "Yes, milk thistle is the traditional favorite and really works."

Thanks to Olive and Leppert for their $.02, and we hope that J.H.'s friend is feeling better soon.

Do you have comments, questions or suggestions that you'd like to share? We're always interested to know what you're thinking. Just click into the HSI Forum at www.healthiertalk.com and add your voice to this and other health care discussions.

To Your Good Health,

Jenny Thompson
Health Sciences Institute

Sources:

- "Bacteria Defies Last-Resort Antibiotic" Nature News Service, 7/26/02
- "Shield Yourself From Deadly "Smart Bugs" HSI Members Alert, 8/1/01

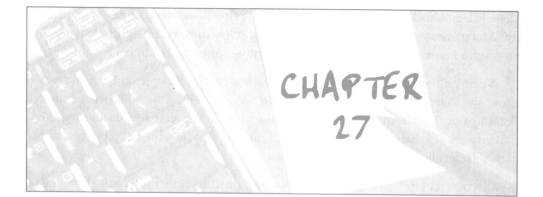

Going Hollywood: Celebrities pitching pharmaceutical drugs

First ran 8/12/2002

When you tune in to a television talk show you expect to see celebrities pitching their latest movie, book or TV show. What you may not expect is that a celebrity might casually plug a product without mentioning that, oh by the way, they've received payment in return for their pitch.

But that's exactly what's going on quite frequently these days. And guess what they're pitching? You get bonus points if you said, "prescription drugs."

The perfect pitch

Yesterday I picked up the New York Times to find an article revealing this clever, albeit shocking, new advertising scheme that drug companies have dreamed up. Among those who are playing the parts of celebrities with helpful medical advice are Lauren Bacall, Kathleen Turner and Rob Lowe, to name a few.

When Lauren Bacall was recently interviewed by Matt Lauer on the Today show, she shared a story about a friend who was blinded by macular degeneration. Pointing out that the disease can strike quickly and unexpectedly, Bacall suggested that viewers see their doctors to get tested for this disease which can be treated with a drug called Visudyne.

It's a perfect pitch: state the health problem, instill a little motivating fear, suggest an action to take, then name the miracle remedy to ask for.

What Bacall didn't tell viewers is that she received a payment from Novartis, the maker of Visudyne, to tell this story. And, according to the article, Matt Lauer and others at NBC were aware of the payment, but they never informed viewers either.

Dr. Joseph Turow, a communications professor at the University of Pennsylvania, feels that this sort of subtle pitch is at best "problematic," and at worst, unethical. He told the New York Times, "When it comes to issues of health, particularly medicines, transparency is an ethical concern. People should be clear about the reasons they are making certain recommendations."

Playing one on TV

But sometimes actors are not recommending a drug. Rather, they're "raising awareness" of a disease or a disorder that is—surprise!—commonly treated with a prescription drug.

Actor Noah Wyle, who plays the part of Dr. John Carter on the NBC hospital drama "ER," appeared twice on the Today show to help raise awareness of post-traumatic stress disorder (PTSD). In both cases it was made clear that he was being paid by Pfizer, the sponsor of the PTSD campaign. The resulting interviews (again, with Matt Lauer) were unintentionally hilarious, with Lauer asking Wyle health-related questions as if he were a doctor, instead of someone who makes a living by pretending to be a doctor.

At no point in either interview was any mention made of the antidepressant drug that's widely prescribed to treat PTSD: Zoloft, which is produced by Pfizer. So Wyle wasn't selling the drug, he was selling the disorder. It's as if Pfizer was saying, "You just get them into the doctor's office, Noah. We'll take care of the drug sale."

Selling the disorder is a booming business in Hollywood. There are already a number of agencies that specialize in manufacturing health-related "education" campaigns, matching movie stars with drug companies. The star gets a lucrative endorsement deal with the appealing cache of being associated with a campaign to bring hope to the afflicted. The agency gets their slice of the deal, of course. And the drug company gets a famous and trustworthy, smiling face who delivers the "awareness" message: "You might have this problem. Go see your doctor. He has a prescription drug for it."

Not the best system

Lauren Bacall and Noah Wyle may be very sincere individuals who dedicate themselves tirelessly to assist those with macular degeneration and PTSD. But I'm guessing that's probably not the case. It's more likely that they've been persuaded by managers and agents to make some hay out of their fame and trade their public images for an easy payday.

It's a numbers game. If the drug companies fill doctors' waiting rooms with patients responding to "awareness campaigns," they have more chances to sell more drugs. Are the patients being served? For the pharmaceutical giants, that would seem to be an afterthought. With the billions they spend on advertising and endorsement deals with celebrities, they're forced into a bottom line mentality that focuses on two goals: prescribe, and, whenever possible, overprescribe.

There's a fine line between being reasonably cautious about your health, and being hypercautious. Hypercaution, dressed up with the glamour of movie stars, seems to be what the drug companies are aiming for.

...and another thing

In an e-Alert I sent you last week ("The power of the single word" 8/8/02) I told you about a new study that confirms previous tests that show how the intake of dietary folate may reduce your homocysteine level.

While writing that one, I was reminded of another small study I'd come across last month about folate and colon cancer.

Researchers at the Royal Victoria Hospital in Belfast, Northern Ireland, studied the effects of a folate supplement on 6 subjects, each of who had recurrent colon polyps. The supplement—2 milligrams of folate—was taken daily for 3 months.

The Belfast team evaluated samples from all of the subjects to determine if cells from the lining of the rectum were dividing and multiplying. The subjects who took folate showed a reduction of cell proliferation. After the folate intake period had finished, however, cell proliferation returned to normal.

The conclusion: for people who are at risk of the disease, a daily folate sample may help keep colon cancer proliferation in check.

One important note: the authors of the study warned that consuming too much folate may be harmful for people with advanced cancer, or those who are taking medication for epilepsy. Which brings us back to my recommendation from last week: most of us can get all the folate we need from natural dietary sources, such as spinach, leafy green vegetables, asparagus, beans and chickpeas.

To Your Good Health,

Jenny Thompson
Health Sciences Institute

Sources:

- "Heartfelt Advice, Hefty Fees" New York Times, 8/11/02
- "Folate Supplement May Reduce Colon Cancer Risk" Reuters Health, 7/18/02

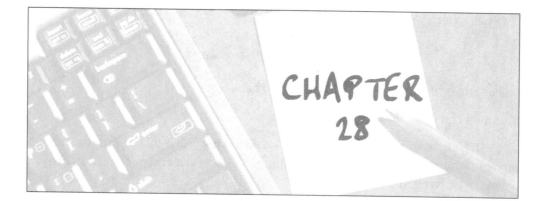

Greasing the skids: Fast food that's good for your heart?

First ran 9/9/2002

Warning! If you're planning to sue McDonald's on the basis that no one ever informed you that its food may be harmful to your health, immediately scroll down to "...and another thing" because here's a news flash: McDonald's fried foods—yes, it's true—may be harmful to your health!

You probably heard the news last week that McDonald's is crowing proudly about its new cooking oil that reduces trans-fatty acids (TFA) by almost half. So that's good, right? Trans-fatty acids are, nutritionally speaking, the fast track to heart disease. So knocking out half the trans-fatty acids makes McDonald's French fries half as dangerous as before, right?

In two words: no way.

Although McDonald's would love you to believe it.

An oil change and a marketing tune up

First, let's get one thing straight: McDonald's is not a fast food joint. It's a "quick service restaurant" (QSR). That's according to the press release McDonald's distributed last week to announce they would begin using a new oil to deep fry French fries, filet-o-fish sandwiches, chicken McNuggets, etc. The "oil change" will be phased in between October 2002, and February 2003, and will reduce trans-fatty acids by 48%, and saturated fat by 16%. Meanwhile, polyunsaturated fat will get a 167% boost.

McDonald's claims that, "While the total fat content in the fries remains unchanged, health experts agree that reducing TFAs and saturates while increasing polyunsaturates is beneficial to heart health." That's sort of like saying, if you reduce your ice cream intake from 5 gallons per week to 2.5 gallons, it's beneficial to your health. Statistically it would probably be true, but it certainly wouldn't be time to go around bragging about your new "healthy" reduced ice cream diet.

The four words that jump out from the McDonald's comment above are the last four—the four they want to leave you with: "beneficial to heart health." That's the central idea this "new oil" campaign would most like to plant in the minds of consumers. "Let's go to McDonald's—I heard their fries are beneficial to heart health!"

In fact, health experts do agree that reducing TFAs is beneficial to heart health. But reducing it by half barely even begins to benefit your heart.

Trans-fatty lowdown

Trans-fats are created by the hydrogenation of vegetable oil—a process that gives the oil a longer shelf life and makes it less greasy. These two qualities also make hydrogenated vegetable oil an appealing and economical choice for "quick service" restaurants and snack foods such as cookies, crackers and chips. Unfortunately, many studies over the past decade have shown trans-fatty acids to be associated with artery damage and a high risk of heart disease.

In an e-Alert I sent you last month ("The New Big Oil" 8/20/02) I told you about a report submitted in July by a National Academy of Sciences panel that attempted to set a safe intake level for trans-fatty acids. The report confirmed previous findings about the relationship of trans-fatty acids and the risk of heart disease, and concluded with a recommendation that cannot be misinterpreted, no matter how you spin the details or rework the words of "health experts." The panel's conclusion: "the only safe intake of trans-fat is zero."

And if that comment doesn't slam the door on the "deep-fried" question, consider the announcement made this past spring by researchers at Stockholm University who studied the effects of high-heat cooking on carbohydrate-rich foods (see the e-Alert "Feeling the Heat" 6/6/02). Among their unsettling conclusions, the Stockholm team found that deep-frying of potato products causes a spontaneous creation of acrylamide, a compound that the International Agency for Research on Cancer and the U.S. government both classify as "probably carcinogenic to humans."

Don't Supersize the fries

Ann Rusniak, R.D., is McDonald's Corporation Chief Nutritionist, and that can't be an easy job. For one thing, people probably think she's kidding when she tells them what her job title is. And for another thing, she has to make statements like this one (that appears under her name on McDonald's web site) and keep a straight face:

"A majority of nutrition professionals have maintained that McDonald's food can be a part of a healthy diet based on the sound nutrition principles of balance, variety and moderation."

Unless Ms. Rusniak is counting every single McDonald's employee (in more than 30,000 restaurants world wide) as "nutrition professionals," there's no way that a majority of genuine nutrition professionals could possibly maintain any of that baloney.

But for a moment let's give Ms. Rusniak and McDonald's the benefit of the doubt. After all, they have gone to the trouble of making the transition to a lower trans-fat cooking oil. They're at least TRYING to make their fried foods healthier, right? Unfortunately we can't answer that one yet because McDonald's still hasn't revealed the specifics about their new oil. They've cut the trans-fat by half, but at what cost? History has shown that when you tinker with the chemistry of cooking oils you inevitably come up with both plusses and minuses. So right now we can only wonder if this new oil might begin creating health problems that won't come to light until another 3 billion customers are served.

...and another thing

In an e-Alert I sent you last week ("Sugar in the Morning, Sugar in the Evening..." 9/4/02) I was pleased to introduce a new herbal product called Glucotor that helps manage blood sugar levels and additional health problems associated with diabetes.

I've received a large response from that e-Alert, including a number of questions sent in by HSI members. Glucotor was formulated by HSI Panelist Jon Barron, so I asked Jon to answer a couple of questions I received.

The first e-mail comes from an HSI member named Joshua who wrote: "Nowhere in this e-alert does it mention which type of diabetics were tested. Was it type 1 or was it type 2, as in most testing? My wife is a type 1 diabetic, and I would like to know if this formula would be effective in type 1 cases."

Jon's reply:

"It was tested on Type II diabetes. However, since it helps dramatically lessen how much sugar enters the body, and since it helps rebuild beta cells in the pancreas, it theoretically could be of some benefit in Type I diabetes too. It does not, though, address the underlying cause of Type I diabetes.

"Doing the whole Baseline of Health program, however, is likely to have much greater impact since it helps tremendously with autoimmune disorders, the primary suspected cause of Type I diabetes. And using digestive enzymes both with meals and between meals significantly reduces Circulating Immune Complexes, a primary contributing factor in autoimmune disorders.

"If you have not already done so, you might want to read 'Lessons from the

Miracle Doctors,' which will explain the program in more detail. You can download a free copy at www.jonbarron.com"

Another HSI member named Jim had this question: "Re: Glucotor, can this be used as a preventative product? Over the last several years I notice my Glucose reading is on the edge or just over the edge of normal. It would seem this product could be one that pushes that range well back into normal."

Jon's response:

"YES! Absolutely. I actually think that's a much more important use of the product. I use one or two capsules a day myself whenever I eat high glycemic foods to smooth out the effect on the body."

These are just two of the many responses I received about the Glucotor e-Alert. To find out more about how Glucotor may be able to help balance your blood sugar, visit the Healing America web site at www.northernnutrition.healingamerica.com).

Meanwhile, my thanks to the many who have responded to the e-Alert, and to Jon for fielding these important questions.

And to McDonald's, for worrying about our heart health.

To Your Good Health,

Jenny Thompson
Health Sciences Institute

Sources:

- "McDonald's USA Announces Significant Reduction of Trans Fatty Acids with Improved Cooking Oil" McDonald's Press Release, 9/3/02

- "McDonald's New Recipe Lowers Goo for Arteries" New York Times, 9/4/02

- "McDonald's Slims Down Spuds" CNN, 9/3/02

- "Trans Fatty Acid Reduction Is a Major Step Toward the Goal of Eliminating Trans Fats From Cooking Oil" Bob Langert, mcdonalds.com

- "Taking Another Look at McDonald's" Ann Rusniak, R.D., mcdonalds.com

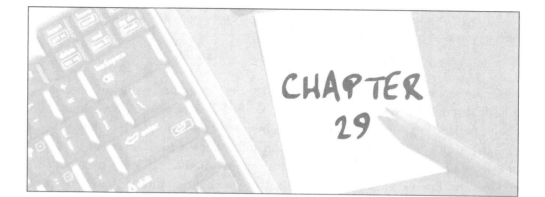

CHAPTER
29

The indelible year: Loss and acute grief

First ran 9/11/2002

I'll be honest, I grappled with how to begin this e-Alert—and how to end it. Because for one year now we've been coping with that thing that's always there, whether we address it directly or not. Everything that's happened in 365 days—all the complex but "normal" passages of life—have, inevitably been measured against a sense of grief, both personal and collective.

Over the past year, I've heard a lot of people talk about the psychological implications of 9/11—the post-traumatic stress disorder, the feelings of loneliness or powerlessness, and the concept of "survivor guilt" that we all suffered as a nation.

But when we think about the impact that grief has on us, we can't overlook the serious physical implications it brings.

Easier said than done.

On the evening of Saturday, November 28, 1942, a fire broke out and spread quickly through a popular Boston nightclub called the Coconut Grove. Almost 500 people perished in the devastating blaze, and it took every firefighter and policeman in the city to deal with the destruction and its aftermath. This event produced one of the first and most influential clinical studies on loss and acute grief. For several months, Erich Lindemann, M.D., a Boston psychiatrist, interviewed survivors and bereaved relatives of the Coconut Grove fire. His report appeared in the "American Journal of Psychiatry" in September, 1944, and included this passage:

"The picture shown by people with acute grief is remarkably uniform. Common to all is the following syndrome: sensations of somatic distress occurring in waves lasting from 20 minutes to an hour at a time, feelings of tightness in the throat, choking with shortness of breath, need for sighing, and an empty feeling in the abdomen, lack of muscular power, and intensive subjective distress described as tension or pain."

Dr. Lindemann clearly understood that grieving carries both an emotional and a physical response. Later studies have come to recognize some of the most common physical reactions associated with grief, such as: listlessness, fatigue, weight loss, irritability, insomnia, loss of appetite, and gastrointestinal complications. On the surface, these may seem like temporary conditions that will disappear as the grieving process runs its course. However, all of them can lead to more serious illnesses.

And while it's really the best thing we could do for ourselves, there's something almost impertinent about suggesting to someone who is grieving to be sure to stay active, get plenty of rest and maintain a nutritious diet.

What you need, when you need it

As Sigmund Freud pointed out in a 1917 essay titled "Mourning and Melancholia" "...after a lapse of time it (grief) will be overcome, and we look upon any interference with it as inadvisable or even harmful."

But until grief is overcome, it's critical that we do whatever we can to limit the long-term impact of grief. Granted, this advice may be better directed to family, friends and co-workers of those who are experiencing grief. So, if someone you care about is grieving, rest assured that you can help.

In terms of specific nutrients, those experiencing grief will benefit from any source that provides high levels of B vitamins—which can be helpful in times of depression and stress, but are also often depleted during those times. In addition to supplements, good dietary sources of vitamin B are: tuna, salmon, avocados, bananas, mangoes, potatoes, broccoli, cauliflower, poultry and meat.

A grieving person may also benefit from additional magnesium in their diet, available through whole grains, nuts and leafy green vegetables.

And to help them manage the psychological impact, there are common herbs like valerian root, chamomile, black cohosh, rosemary, and St. John's wort that can help control the emotional roller coaster.

There's no cure for grief, obviously, but there are ways to address, and even avoid, its physical side effects, until the moment comes when we turn the corner and are ready to embrace life again.

...and another thing

9/11

One year ago today we all stopped in our tracks. We were glued to our televisions and watched, unable to believe what we were seeing, and unable to deny that it was all too real.

At the hour the two planes hit the twin towers, my father was at Newark airport waiting for a flight to New Mexico. I knew he was flying out that morning, but I didn't know when. Was he in the air? Phones everywhere were down so there was no way to reach him, no way to get in touch with the airlines. All I could do, like so many others, was wait. (It was a little more than two hours before I knew my father was home and safe. His flight had never left the ground.)

Next we heard about the Pentagon. Then the crash in Pennsylvania. For the first time in generations, millions of Americans suddenly knew what it was like to live in a country under attack. Was it over? Was it just beginning? Added to this uncertainty was the feeling of futility in being attacked by enemies who vanished at the moment of their victory, making it impossible to fight back. Or so it seemed at the moment. As we now know, a handful of Americans, the passengers of flight 93, were the first to respond...refusing to let the terrorists win the rest of round one.

In many ways all of our lives have returned to normal. Although normal is entirely different now. We have a new and stronger resolve to defend our free society as we continue our response to terror, begun on the morning of 9/11 by the brave passengers of Flight 93, and carried on by each of us throughout this indelible year.

In remembrance,

Jenny Thompson
Health Sciences Institute

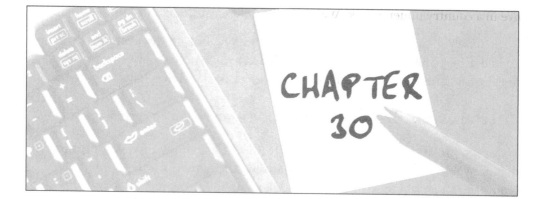

Taking pity: Pharmaceutical companies continue to exploit loopholes

First ran 9/19/2002

Sometimes it seems like international pharmaceutical companies just can't catch a break.

This past June I told you about a couple of tough hits the drug giants recently had to endure. Congress was hounding them with the Greater Access to Affordable Pharmaceuticals Act, designed to close some legal loopholes and make them let go of their stranglehold on expired patents. Then on July 1st, a new set of voluntary guidelines went into effect that called for pharmaceutical salespeople to cut back on the gifts, meals, sports event tickets, "consulting" gigs and other perks they've used to encourage doctors to prescribe their products.

So have you been lying awake at night wondering how in the world these belea-guered drug giants are getting along? Well, don't you worry. They've been doing just fine. Let me bring you up to date about how the poor wretches have been coping.

Extensions that keep on going, and going, and going...

"Pretty in Pink" was the title of the 6/18/02 e-Alert about a tricky little move that drug companies have been using to extend the patents on their premiere, money-making products. And who can blame them for trying? They spend millions, sometimes billions of dollars to produce a best selling product, and then as soon as they get a patent, the generic drug companies start laying plans to move in when the patent expires. At that time, the generic versions of the drug hit the market and the former patent holder can only stand aside as the profits of its former gravy train product start rolling in for someone else.

Did I say, "stand aside"? What I meant to say was: "launch a battalion of attorneys to sniff out and pry open every available loophole." Which is their right, of course. After all, exploiting loopholes is a great American pastime. But when does too much become just way too much? When even the U.S. Senate takes notice.

In June I told you about how a patent holder can claim that its drug has a new use or a newly added chemical property, and based on these claims, the FDA will often grant a patent extension of 30 extra months even though the change in the product may be only superficial. Eli Lilly, for instance, took their superstar workhorse, Prozac, gave it a different color, and under a new name offered it as a relief to premenstrual irritability. And for their efforts they got a big O.K. on that from the FDA.

In the meantime, drug companies also found that they could extend a patent by claiming that the generic manufacturer of the drug had violated a regulation. What specific regulation was being questioned didn't matter because, simply by asserting the claim, a 30-month patent extension was automatically granted. In addition, if a drug company had more than one patent on a drug, they could get more than one extension by making additional claims. That's where the Senate drew a line in the sand and passed a bill designed to cut off the drug companies at only one 30-month extension.

But those drug company lobbyists and legal teams don't go and get all submissive when the Senate says, "Stop." No way. A Senate bill is nothing more than a wake-up call to them.

How many times do I have to tell ya?

The Congressional Budget Office (CBO) has estimated that if the Senate bill becomes a law, it could save consumers as much as $60 billion over the next decade. And the drug companies would still be able to defend their patents. Everyone wins, right? Well, no. Because if you're a pharmaceutical company this is what you hear in that CBO statement: the Senate is allowing consumers to take away $60 billion that is rightfully yours.

But consumers wouldn't be the only winners. A number of large corporations would reap huge financial benefits from the passage of this bill by reducing the cost of company health plans. As a result, some of those corporations lobbied in favor of the legislation. But some of those corporations forgot that they had business partners who were drug companies. Oops.

Georgia-Pacific Paper Company, for instance, was about to conclude a three-year sales deal with Eli Lilly, when it suddenly found that Lilly was not pleased that G-P was a member of Business for Affordable Medicine (BAM). (Affordable medicine! What were they thinking?) Georgia-Pacific saw the light and asked that its name be withdrawn from the BAM web site. Eli Lilly reps denied that they pressured G-P, but admitted that they do have a policy of contacting business partners to "explain" why they don't support the Senate bill.

I can't help but wonder if that "explaining" session might have resembled a scene out of "The Sopranos."

Meanwhile, it must be gratifying to the entire pharmaceutical industry that Verizon Communications, Marriott International and United Parcel Service have all pulled back on their support of Business for Affordable Medicine, as well as the Senate bill. Apparently they just needed the situation "explained" to them.

More to come...

If you'd like to see a list of the companies still requiring further explanation or more details on the pending legislation, you can visit the web site maintained by the Business for Affordable Medicine (bamcoalition.org).

Next week I'll have further reports from the front lines of the drug industry's ongoing battles. I'll give you an update on the Pharmaceutical Research and Manufacturers of America (PhRMA) guidelines that went into effect last summer to govern the relationships between drug companies and physicians. And I'll also tell you the tale of a former senior consultant to the FDA who now claims that the government agency often sacrifices safety for speed in the approval of new drugs, especially when "user fees" are changing hands.

It just keeps getting better and better. Or, rather, worse and worse.

To Your Good Health,

Jenny Thompson
Health Sciences Institute

Sources:

■ "Big Drug Makers' Tactics" the Washington Post, 9/16/02

The drug salesman & the PhRAMA's daughter:
Are new marketing codes for drug companies being followed?

First ran 9/23/2002

Did you hear the one about the PhRMA guidelines?
Last summer I sent you an e-Alert ("Barbarians at the Garden Gate" 6/27/02) about the new marketing code of the Pharmaceutical Research and Manufacturers of America (PhRMA), designed to govern the pharmaceutical industry's relationships with physicians. The sweet ride was over, PhRMA said, because its new set of strict guidelines detailed exactly how far a drug salesperson could go to influence physicians to prescribe, prescribe, prescribe, and (when in doubt) over-prescribe.

But PhRMA is an advocacy group for the drug industry. They have no regulatory power, so the most they can do is to ask salespeople to stick to these guidelines on a voluntary basis.

So how do you suppose that's been working out?

Influence—bought & sold

The new "PhRMA Code on Interactions with Healthcare Professionals" started off with two strikes against it: ten years ago the American Medical Association initiated similar guidelines (which nobody followed); and the PhRMA guidelines are filled with language that provides plenty of loopholes. Under these circumstances, it's easy to imagine how pharmaceutical companies might not be motivated to voluntarily pull back on the methods they've used for many years to influence and persuade their clients.

Even though the new code has been in effect for only two and a half months, the "Newark Star Ledger" decided to get the jump on everyone, reporting that some doctors claim the guidelines are being ignored. For instance, one of the PhRMA rules calls for drug salespeople to treat healthcare providers to only modestly priced meals. But the drug giant GlaxoSmithKline recently booked an expensive French restaurant to host a lecture for doctors from the University of Pennsylvania Hospital.

Similar incidents of other drug companies stepping over the PhRMA guidelines have been reported by doctors at the U. Penn Hospital. And although the Star Ledger highlighted only these isolated events, I believe we'll be hearing similar reports from other sources nationwide. And, really, did we expect not to? The PhRMA guidelines have no teeth. Their primary purpose is public relations: to show the world that the industry is at least making an effort. But while PhRMA is sending a message to the public, I hope the word is getting through to the one group that most needs to hear and understand the concept that influence should not be bought and sold: the doctors.

I'm convinced that the pharmaceutical industry can only be regulated by the health care professionals it serves. When a drug salesperson attempts to influence a doctor with gifts and other perks, there are two parties present at that point of contact. If a doctor accepts the special offers of a salesperson and in return prescribes patent drugs instead of less expensive generic drugs, that doctor is serving himself and the drug company. Meanwhile, his patients—who trust him to provide the best quality care at the lowest cost—are not being served. But if the doctor simply refuses the gifts and perks, then the problem vanishes along with the need for unnecessary regulations. Needless to say, when your doctor prescribes a name brand drug, you should always ask if a generic is available.

Whistle blowing

But I don't want to let the drug companies off the hook here. Time and time again they've demonstrated marketing practices that would make an organized crime boss blush.

In last Thursday's e-Alert ("Taking Pity" 9/19/02) I told you how the drug companies are not above flexing their economic influence and leaning on business partners outside of their industry who might be inclined to support legislation unfavorable to the pharmaceutical conglomerates. Last week I also came across an article with this chilling headline: "Insider: Drug Safety Not FDA Priority." And guess who's right in the middle of this story, doing everything they can to press the FDA to speed along approvals of new drugs while downplaying safety issues. Did you answer "drug companies"? Right on the money!

The "insider" mentioned in the headline is Paul Stolley, M.D., M.P.H., a former FDA advisor who served as an FDA safety-consultant for two years. Now he's blowing the whistle, charging that the drug approval process is heavily influenced by drug companies who pay "product review" fees. Among other claims, Dr. Stolley says that the drug giants fully expect the reviews to speed through as quickly as possible in return for the payment of these fees.

I'm sure this story will soon be followed with additional rebuttals and accusations. So I'll keep watch for further reports, and then I'll bring you a full accounting of Dr. Stolley's insider-insights.

...and another thing

Two weeks ago I sent you an e-Alert ("Greasing the Skids" 9/9/02) about the dangers of trans-fatty acids (TFA) in cooking oil—particularly the types of cooking oil used by fast food restaurants. Coincidentally, that same day an article appeared in the Wall St. Journal about TFA. Here's an email I received from an HSI member named Frank about the WSJ article:

"Could you respond to Steven Milloy's article in the Sept. 9 issue of the 'Wall Street Journal' ('McJunk Science')? Briefly, he says that the available evidence really doesn't substantiate the claim that trans-fatty acids raise the risk of heart disease in humans. He further states that, 'none of the six studies of human populations consuming trans fats come close to linking them with heart disease.'"

To answer Frank's question I would say: "Consider the source."

Steven J. Milloy is an author and a former lobbyist for Phillip Morris Tobacco Company. He has a background in natural science and biostatistics, and in recent years has earned a firebrand reputation for debunking what he calls "junk science." And although I find that I agree with him on some points (for instance: elevated cholesterol doesn't necessarily lead to heart disease), other information I've read forces me to take issue with his opinion on trans-fatty acids.

Following the logic of considering the source, I would rather get my TFA information from someone more like Mary G. Enig, Ph.D, a widely respected nutritionist with a specialty in the nutritional aspects of fats and oils, a Fellow of the American College of Nutrition, and a member of the American Institute of Nutrition. In a decade of research, Dr. Enig has shown that trans-fatty acids consumption results in a number of adverse health effects, including heart disease, obesity, diabetes and even cancer.

Commenting on one of those "six studies in human populations" that he dismissed, Mr. Milloy had this to say about a well-known Harvard study: "My favorite...study that fails to link trans fats with heart disease—one involving 90,000 nurses followed for 20 years—also fails to link total fat intake, saturated-fat intake, animal-fat intake and cholesterol intake with heart disease."

Meanwhile, Dr. Enig says that the Harvard study clearly showed that subjects who developed heart disease had a significantly higher intake of TFA than subjects who never developed heart disease.

So we have a classic "he said—she said." Consider the sources and make your own call.

To Your Good Health,

Jenny Thompson
Health Sciences Institute

Sources:

- "Drug Makers Still Picking up Docs' Tab " the Newark Star-Ledger, 9/4/02

- "FDA Swayed by Drug Industry, Former Insider Charges" Reuters Health, 9/13/02

- "Insider: Drug Safety Not FDA Priority / Does Agency Serve the Public— or the Drug Industry?" WebMD, 9/12/02

- "McJunk Science" Steven Milloy, the Wall Street Journal, 9/9/02

- "Health Risks from Processed Foods and the Dangers of Trans Fats" Dr. Mary Enig Interviewed By Richard A. Passwater, Ph.D. (Dr. Joseph Mercola)

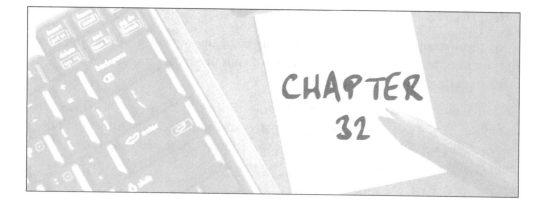

Hear that lonesome whistle blow? Former FDA advisor makes startling claims

First ran 10/02/2002

It can't be easy to be an executive at a giant pharmaceutical corporation. On one hand, you manufacture products that promise to improve the health of your customers. On the other hand, you have the relentless bottom line pressures of a complex and enormous corporate structure in which significant profit growth is mandatory.

Every company has interests that are sometimes at odds with one another, and settling differences calls for compromise. But the pharmaceutical industry is one of those businesses where the quality of the product absolutely must not be compromised. That's the theory anyway.

So if you're an executive with a huge drug company, on which side do you draw your bottom line? On the side of the safety of your product? Or on the side of profit margins and stockholder interests?

I'd like to think I know where I would draw the line. But I'm also sure I wouldn't last more than 20 minutes as a drug company executive. Because again and again we see the evidence that those executives sometimes turn their heads and let the chips (and the health of consumers) fall where they may.

Time is money

Last week in an e-Alert about the recent guidelines established for drug company salespeople ("The Drug Salesman and the PhRMA's Daughter" 9/23/02), I told you about a former FDA advisor who now claims that the drug approval process is heavily influenced by drug companies who pay "product review" fees. I told you I would follow this story for later developments, and, just as I expected, more damaging information has come along.

In a nutshell, here's how a new drug gets approved. After Drug Company XYZ applies to have a new drug investigated, FDA representatives become involved in determining the structure of human trials. Trial data is reviewed by FDA scientists and sometimes sent to an advisory committee. XYZ is sometimes invited to present its pitch for the drug at a public meeting. When the FDA determines that the drug is safe, it makes a final approval and tells XYZ what information must appear on the drug label. This process often takes up to two and a half years. That's 2+ years of zero return on a drug that may represent millions of dollars in investment. And that just won't do.

So in 1993 Congress gave the drug companies a gift called the Prescription Drug User Fee Act (PDUFA) that allows the FDA to charge the drug companies a product review fee. In exchange, the FDA promises a speedy review process for new drug applications. On average, the approval process now takes about half as long as it used to. But is that enough time to determine the safety of a new drug? Believe it or not, there are still many people out there who are completely comfortable with putting their personal safety in the hands of the FDA.

Safety takes a back seat

Paul Stolley, M.D., M.P.H., is a former chairman of preventive medicine at the University of Maryland, and served as an FDA advisor and safety-consultant for two years. Last month, the British Medical Journal reported on comments made by Dr. Stolley which give details and confirmation to what was already suspected: that, in Dr. Stolley's words, "The FDA has a philosophy that innovation is to be worshipped and drugs are to be speeded through as quickly as possible. This philosophy holds that people who worry about safety and risk are holding up new ideas and keeping medicine from a needy public."

This charge is firmly backed up by the example of two high profile recalls of drugs that enjoyed the FDA's fast track approval process. Baycol, a cholesterol lowering drug manufactured by Bayer AG, and a GlaxoSmithKline Plc irritable bowel syndrome drug called Lotronex were both withdrawn when linked to the death of patients. In fact, Dr. Stolley's falling out with FDA executives began with his warnings about the safety of Lotronex—warnings that unfortunately went unheeded.

Amazingly, the FDA recently recommended to allow Lotronex—a known killer—back on the market under a risk-management program that would limit its use to patients who suffer from severe irritable bowel problems. Dr. Stolley agrees that some drugs should be allowed under risk-management programs, but that Lotronex should not because its complications are so unpredictable.

What haste makes

In the British Medical Journal, Dr. Stolley noted that, "In the last decade we have seen an unusual number of withdrawals soon after approval."

Last month the U.S. General Accounting Office (GAO) officially confirmed that charge. Congress recently asked the GAO to investigate links between the shortened drug approval period and the rates of drugs recalled from the market. In its report, released on September 22, the GAO stated that since the enactment of PDUFA, the percentage of drugs withdrawn from the market for safety-related reasons has been steadily on the rise.

Clearly, millions of people assume that the FDA is watching out for their best interests. They trust the FDA to thoroughly test new drugs, and then withhold any drug that's dangerous, or fully report on the adverse side effects of drugs that are deemed ready for market. If the FDA is incapable of managing these tasks quickly, then they owe it to the public to let them know. Maybe drugs that receive the PDUFA treatment should be labeled as "Fast Track Approved." But would anyone really believe in the safety of the approval process if those three words were printed across the top of their prescription?

What Congress will do in response to the GAO report is not clear. I'll watch the news wires and keep you posted. Meanwhile, we now have confirmation of what most of us have known for a long time—that we should never assume that an FDA approval equals safety.

...and another thing

And now for something completely different—a good word about the FDA.

No kidding.

This week, the Food and Drug Administration began the first in a series of meetings to plan research designed to understand what can be done to reduce or eliminate acrylamide from cooked foods.

Last spring I sent you an e-Alert ("Feeling the Heat" 6/6/02) about research from Stockholm University in Sweden with a warning that a carcinogen called acrylamide is created when foods (especially carbohydrates) are cooked at high temperatures. This alarming study was quickly followed up over the summer with similar studies in Norway, Switzerland and the United Kingdom—all of them drawing virtually the same conclusions.

The preliminary results from the Stockholm study showed that the highest levels of acrylamide occur in potato products, with bread containing somewhat lower levels, and breakfast cereals containing the least. This news, coupled with what we already know about the trans-fatty acids in oil used for deep frying, would have to qualify fast food French fries as just about the worst thing you can possibly eat.

But fries are not the only culprits. The recent studies have named names: potato chips, crackers, pastries, and powdered coffee all contain high levels of acrylamide, while fried fish and fried chicken contain somewhat lower amounts.

The FDA is working closely with the World Health Organization on this project. They hope to have final recommendations ready by the early part of 2004. And what do we do until then? An FDA spokesman suggested this revolutionary concept: we should eat a balanced diet with plenty of fruits and vegetables and lay off the fried foods.

Hmmm...an unconventional bit of conventional wisdom from the FDA. Is there a full moon?

To Your Good Health,

Jenny Thompson
Health Sciences Institute

Sources:

- "FDA Swayed by Drug Industry, Former Insider Charges" Reuters Health, 9/11/02

- "Insider: Drug Safety Not FDA Priority" Daniel DeNoon, Web MD, 9/12/02

- "FDA Fees may be Tied to Drug Recalls / Government Report Questions Safety Review System" Reuters, 9/24/02

- "FDA Launches Plan to Reduce Acrylamides in Foods" Alicia Ault, Reuters, 9/30/02

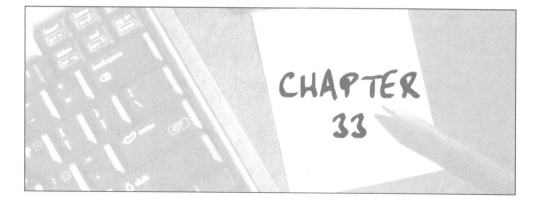

CHAPTER 33

Physician, hear thyself: Insurance industry premiums and the right to care

First ran 10/10/2002

The other day I received an e-mail that was a little upsetting. It came from an e-Alert reader who had taken my frequent references to homocysteine to heart and asked her doctor to check her homocysteine level—which is a good idea for anyone concerned about reducing the risk of heart disease, heart attack and stroke. As I've often mentioned, your homocysteine level more accurately reveals the risk of heart related disorders than a cholesterol test.

So what could be the problem with a homocysteine test? You draw blood, send it off to the lab, and wait for results. Simple enough. But sometimes the simplest things can become unnecessarily complicated when outside pressures come into play.

Getting tagged

To ensure this reader's privacy, I'm not going to give her real name. We'll call her Tracy. And here's part of her e-mail:

"I was at my doctor's office the other day for my annual exam and asked if I could have my homocysteine level checked. She said she would highly recommend against this because, since I have no other "risk factors" for heart disease, my health insurance premiums would rise when they see a test for homocysteine. She also said what good would it do since I already take B vitamins, I exercise six days a week, I'm thin and lean, and I'm premenopausal.

"Normally, my response would have been that since I am on my husband's group plan at work my premiums won't go up. But then I thought that since my husband is going to retire in a few years and I'll have to get my own, non-group insurance, that maybe I would be tagged for higher insurance premiums because of this test. Have you ever heard of this? Do you have any comments on this?"

Comments? You know I do!

Something fishy

I rarely discuss the insurance industry in the e-Alert. Insurance is an important tangent to health care, but it's outside the scope of our primary mission at HSI. And besides, I have my hands full with two other hot buttons: the pharmaceutical industry and the FDA.

That said, I'll push this uncustomary button, and make a couple of observations.

Like the pharmaceutical companies, insurance companies are in business for one reason: to make money. So while we'd like to think that they care about our health as much as we do, it simply isn't true. To them our health is a business and our doctors are de facto employees. When you look at it that way, it makes sense that health insurance providers offer incentives to doctors who call for a low number of surgeries and special screenings for their patients. (That probably includes homocysteine screening.) They simply found a way to make their "employees" focus on their bottom line.

Now I don't know Tracy's doctor, she may be a wonderful physician who genuinely had Tracy's best interests in mind. But there is a chance that she was motivated by a concern that was in the insurance company's best interests, not Tracy's. Which, to my mind, violates the doctor-patient relationship plain and simple. When you walk into that office, you have a right to think the doctor is working for YOU while you're there, not Acme Insurance.

Granted, Tracy does not appear to be in a high-risk group for heart disorders. But people outside the normal risk groups suffer from ailments of every kind every day. Is it possible that by getting the test, Tracy's insurance coverage would be "tagged" for higher premiums? I don't know enough about the inner workings of the insurance companies but it certainly sounds like a common practice. But this is a simple blood test. If the test involved an elaborate procedure or a hospital stay, I might buy the tagging story. But raising premiums in response to a simple blood test—and not even considering the results? Frankly, that sounds fishy.

Getting all histrionic about it

Doctors are revered in our society. And they should be. They have a tremendously difficult job to do. And without a doubt, the good ones are worth their weight in gold. But anytime you feel a doctor is not adequately serving your health needs, you have to stand up for yourself and insist on being well served. Of course, this is often easier said than done.

Tracy's story reminded me of an experience of my own. A few months ago I had some vision problems—headaches and trouble focusing. I hadn't had an eye exam in years, so I went to my primary care physician and asked him to refer me to an ophthalmologist. Which he did. And fortunately my problem turned out to be a simple case of eyestrain.

Then, a couple of months later, I developed a severe sore throat. I found it difficult to swallow and my throat was closing up at night. When it became unbearable, I called my doctor. He was out of town, but his receiving nurse scheduled me to see another doctor. When I went in for my appointment, the substitute physician looked over my medical history file and asked about my recent complaint about declining vision. Then he floored me with this casual statement: "That was a bit histrionic, wasn't it?"

No. It was not even remotely histrionic. I was having eye problems and I sought help. But with this comment he revealed his attitude toward his patients' health needs. In effect he was saying: "You exaggerate. You're fine. Don't trust yourself. And don't bother me with your problems."

Thinking about this experience later, I wondered about his other patients and what sort of treatment they regularly receive. Then I imagined someone like my grandmother—someone who had a mild personality and a trusting nature—and how someone like that would be intimidated and, as a result, poorly served by this insensitive doctor.

As many of us do, I let my health problem go on too long before I called for an appointment. I can only imagine that the regular patients of that substitute doctor wait even longer than most people—not wanting to be thought of as hypochondriacs or be labeled as histrionic.

I hope that the next time Tracy gets a check up she'll insist on the homocysteine test. If anyone else has had an experience similar to Tracy's, or if their insurance policies have been tagged for increased premiums in response to a homocysteine test, I'd very much like to hear about it. Because you have every right to expect a "can do" attitude from your doctor when it comes to something as important and the health of your heart.

...and another thing

No doubt you've heard the phrase "the cure is worse than the disease." To that we can now add a new homily: "the prevention is worse than the disease." In at least one case anyway.

This was my reaction to an astonishing article from the Belfast Telegraph sent to me by an HSI member named Michael. A Queen's University study in Ulster, Ireland, found that women with a family history of breast or ovarian cancer have an extremely high lifetime risk of developing those cancers. The researchers estimate that one in 500 women are in this dangerous risk group. Their solution: to prevent cancer, these women should have their breasts and ovaries removed.

One of the researchers, Dr. Paul Harkin, cleared up a key point, stating, "It's important to emphasize that the choice lies with the women themselves."

What a relief! I was afraid he was going to say it was mandatory.

I searched around the Internet, but couldn't find a full report of the study available. I just wanted to check and see if there were any female scientists involved in this study. I can't help but think that the answer to that is probably, "no."

Gentlemen, let's hope these scientists don't conduct similar studies on people who have a family history of prostate or testicular cancers.

To Your Good Health,

Jenny Thompson
Health Sciences Institute

Sources:

- "Drastic Cure for Cancer" Nigel Gould, the Belfast Telegraph, 9/27/02

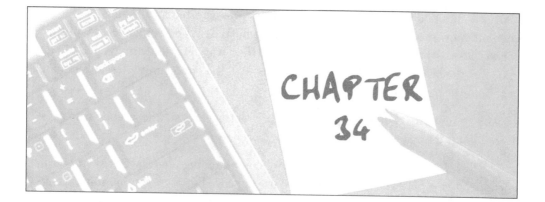

Compounding the issue: Unbalanced reporting on the compounding pharmaceutical industry

First ran 10/15/2002

Maybe you heard the same program I heard yesterday morning on National Public Radio about a recent series of articles that appeared in the Kansas City Star. Under the title, "Rx for Disaster," two veteran KC Star journalists concluded a six-month investigation with a wide ranging report on the dangers and drawbacks of drug compounding. Unfortunately, NPR completely ignored the many benefits of drug compounding. Which is certainly in keeping with the tone of the Star articles, which are little more than a thinly veiled attack.

On one hand, I can forgive the Star reporters for their lack of balance. In August,

2001, a compounding pharmacist in Kansas City was arrested for diluting a chemotherapy mixture, severely compromising the potency of as many as 150 intravenous doses. The pharmacist, Robert R. Courtney, was apparently motivated to endanger the lives of dozens of cancer patients with the opportunity to reap a personal profit of over half a million dollars.

As a community, Kansas City was justifiably outraged. And as someone who cares deeply about the state of healthcare, I am outraged, too.

But that doesn't give NPR license to paint compounding pharmacists as stubborn, uncooperative rebels who simply refuse to use approved drugs. Compounding pharmacy exists as a practice to provide much needed solutions for patients with unique medication requirements. And the NPR report completely failed to acknowledge that critical function.

More than counting pills

Imagine that you had a child with a history of life-threatening allergic reactions. Your child develops a raging infection, which requires treatment with a specific class of antibiotic. The problem is, that antibiotic contains yellow dye #5—a substance that you know would induce a severe reaction in your child. What would you do?

Or, say you suffer from an extremely rare condition that is controlled by a specific prescription drug. But the patent expires, and the pharmaceutical company decides that there isn't enough demand for the drug to justify the expense of a patent renewal and continued production. You need the medicine to manage your symptoms—but now the drug will no longer be available. What options do you have?

Both of these situations present formidable obstacles. But in both cases a solution can be found through a compounding pharmacy.

Compounding pharmacists don't just count out and measure mass-produced drugs as most pharmacists do. Compounders work with your doctor to create a medicine that best fits your specific needs. Ingredients, dosage, concentration, delivery method, flavoring—all of these variables are within the control of the prescribing physician and compounder. For example, a compounding pharmacist can combine two medications into one pill, or formulate some medications into lotions, eye drops, lip balms, nebulizer solutions, or suppositories. They give you options where otherwise you would have none.

An exacting science

Despite the slanted focus of the NPR story, compounding is not just a matter of convenience or preference. In many cases, compounding comes to the rescue in life-threatening situations. For instance, many critically ill patients in hospice care rely on compounded medications because they are unable to swallow pills.

And don't believe anyone who describes a compounding pharmacist as just any old Joe playing mad scientist with controlled substances. We're talking about licensed, educated pharmacists—professionals with years of training. They cannot dispense any medications, compounded or otherwise, without a doctor's prescription. In fact, doctors are the ones who usually initiate the compounding order, asking the pharmacists to formulate the medication according to precise specifications.

Also, all of the ingredients used by compounders are approved drugs listed in the U.S. Pharmacopoeia National Formulary (USP/NF), an encyclopedia of each drug approved by the U.S. Pharmaceutical Convention. So for those of you that are reassured by regulation, you can be sure that there's plenty of it here already (and I mean plenty).

Bathwater goes out–baby stays in

The portrayal of compounding pharmacists as loose cannons running amok is unfair. The reporters of the Kansas City Star have been diligent in running down the details of mistakes and abuses that have occurred among a handful of compounders nationwide. And without question, it's hurtful and sometimes tragic when mistakes are made in any healthcare field. But this is not a situation that's unique to compound pharmacy. Every year, thousands of patients are harmed (sometimes fatally) by health providers who make mistakes using standard prescription drugs.

Our hearts go out to the Kansas City cancer patients who, while fighting for their lives, discovered that the pure greed of a single individual made their fight just that much harder. There's no excuse in the world for that. But there's also no reason to set off on a witch hunt, branding all compounding pharmacists as negligent and dangerous.

...and another thing

Time and again, you've heard the mantra from me and many of my colleagues: The research on natural products is limited because without the ability to patent them, there simply isn't enough profit potential for the big drug companies.

Well, we weren't just whistling Dixie.

HSI Panelist, Allan Spreen, M.D., recently sent me the following commentary on an article he found which sheds light on profit margins that would make even Donald Trump blush.

"I just ran into a report generated by the Life Extension Foundation, the non-profit research organization. In their October 2002 edition of Life Extension magazine they list the cost of the key ingredients of many popular prescription drugs. The antibiotic Keflex, for instance, costs a total of $1.88 for enough of the active ingredient to make 100 of the 250 milligram tablets. The amount that consumers pay for 100 tablets: $157.39 (an 8,372% mark-up).

"Prilosec, the ulcer 'wonder drug,' lists a consumer price of $360.97 for 100 of the 20 milligram tabs—the active ingredient costs the drug company $0.52 (a 69,417% mark-up).

"Not many drug classes are immune. Norvasc, a blood pressure drug, has a consumer price of $188.29 for 100 of the 10 milligram tabs, while the active ingredient cost is $0.14 (a 134,493% mark-up). Prozac (ever heard of that one?) gets into the fun stuff: 100 of the 20 milligram tabs is listed at a consumer price of $247.47, while the active ingredient costs...get ready...$0.11 (224,973% mark-up).

"Now that you need Xanax to assimilate the above numbers, let's see what you pay for it: $136.79 for 100 of the 1 milligram tabs, while the active ingredient cost is 2.4 cents (569,958% mark-up).

"I readily admit that drug companies have other expenses: research & development, packaging, marketing, delivery, product liability, FDA approvals of course, and more, I'm sure. But if you'll guarantee me a captive audience of millions of people having no choice (in their minds) but to buy your product, and permit me to sell your product for a 500,000% mark-up, then I'll pay the additional expenses without a single complaint..."

To Your Good Health,

Jenny Thompson
Health Sciences Institute

Sources:

- "Rx for Disaster" Mark Morris, Jill Toyoshiba, Kansas City Star, 10/6—10/8/02

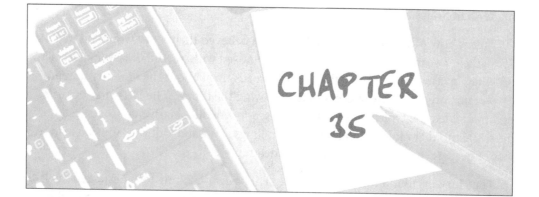

CHAPTER
35

Forcing choices: FDA regulations designed to protect may not be

First ran 11/06/2002

There are few things more infuriating than a bureaucratic system that's designed to protect, but because of a misguided sense of purpose, ends up "protecting" people from the things they need the most.

Confused priorities

Imagine yourself in this scenario: Your child is sick. His doctor offers a treatment that you find unacceptable. So you do some research and find a doctor who has developed a treatment that you feel is right for your child. Could it be simpler? You make your choice and live with the results.

This is how Michael and Raphaele Horwin believed their story would be told. In 1998, their 2 year-old son Alexander was diagnosed with, medulloblastoma—a fast-growing, invasive brain tumor that easily spreads throughout the nervous system. Two brain surgeries were successful in removing the tumor. The Horwins' doctors recommended the typical chemotherapy used for medulloblastoma—an extremely harsh chemo that often damages the heart, lungs, liver and kidneys, and can lead to loss of hearing, further cancers and even death.

The Horwins found this unacceptable. They began looking for alternate treatments and soon located a doctor named Stanislaw Burzynski whose Houston clinic had successfully treated several children with cancer, including medulloblastoma. Burzynski's unconventional treatment used synthetic peptides, purported to "switch off" cancer genes. And although Burzynski's treatments were controversial, they were part of an FDA-approved clinical trial.

But there were two problems. First: The FDA guidelines stipulated that a patient such as Alexander could only receive Burzynski's treatment if he had already been given an "approved" chemotherapy, and the chemo had been ineffective in curbing the cancer. The second problem was presented by Alexander's oncologists. The Horwins got a jolt when they discovered that they had no choice in the matter of Alexander's chemotherapy treatments. The oncologists informed them that, if necessary, they could forcibly remove Alexander to administer the chemo.

Hemmed in by laws and regulations designed to "protect" kids like Alexander, the Horwins reluctantly agreed to begin chemotherapy. After three cycles of the treatments, a CT scan showed that a large number of new tumors had developed. At this point Alexander became eligible for the treatment at the Burzynski clinic, but his cancer was too far advanced. Alexander died three weeks later.

Charlatans in sheep's clothing

The FDA regulations that prohibited the Horwins from seeking treatment for Alexander from Stanislaw Burzynski were designed to "protect" the Horwins and others like them from unscrupulous charlatans who would charge an exorbitant price for an unproven treatment.

Exorbitant price? Alexander's medical bill totaled almost a quarter of a million dollars.

Unproven treatment? Oncologists assured the Horwins that the chemotherapy they administered to Alexander (called CCG-9921) was "state-of-the-art." But after Alexander's death, the Horwins discovered that over a period of more than 20 years, numerous studies in medical journals had reported that this chemo was known to cause dementia, seizures and death. In fact, one study was discontinued when the children's tumors were discovered spreading rather than decreasing. Furthermore, CCG-9921 has been approved by the FDA to treat adults, but its use with children is considered to be "experimental." And yet, in spite of its horrendous track record, CCG-9921 is still being prescribed (or in the case of the Horwins: forced) to treat children with medullablastoma.

So who are the charlatans? Imagine the answer you might get if you asked the Horwins that question. The big difference here, of course, is that charlatans can't force you to use their treatments on your child.

Who controls your healthcare choices?

Based on the notion that the judgment of parents can't be trusted, government regulations forced Alexander Horwin into the harshest imaginable chemotherapy. If the Horwin's had been free to pursue the Burzynski treatments, they could not have possibly done any worse than the government did. But could they have saved Alexander's life? Unfortunately, they'll never know.

Without question, there are true charlatans out there who would prey on desperate people, bilking them of their savings while convincing them that a bogus therapy might save their lives, or the lives of their children. But this is what thorough research and background checks are for. And I would much rather place my faith in each individual's personal judgment before I placed my faith in a bloated bureaucracy, willing to restrict everyone's right to choose in order to protect a few of us from making bad choices.

...and another thing

Last week, I told you about my lunch with an old friend whose doctor was "threatening" her with a prescription for statin drugs ("The Light at the End of the Tunnel Vision" 10/31/02). Let me tell you, after listening to this, it was amazing I was able to eat lunch at all, since I found I was biting my tongue the whole time.

And that happens a lot.

While it's easy for me to share important health information with over 125,000 of you every day through this e-Alert, it can be hard to talk about some of these issues with my friends and family. Sometimes they just don't want to hear it and look at me like I'm a relentless "health nut." Other times, I may not even know what health problems they're facing. So while I could send information that would absolutely help them, I wouldn't necessarily know what to send.

So I take the easy way out. I usually end up encouraging everyone I know to sign up for the e-Alert and just ask them to read it for a few weeks.

To Your Good Health,

Jenny Thompson
Health Sciences Institute

Sources:

- "War on Cancer: Why does the FDA Deny Access to Alternative Cancer Treatments?" Michael Horwin, California Western Law Review, V. 38, No. 1, Fall, 2001
- "FDA Forces Fatal Chemo on Kids" Kristen Philipkoski, wired.com, 10/15/02
- "Parents Fight FDA to Save Son" Lynn Burke, wired.com, 7/18/00
- "Medulloblastoma" brain-tumor.net

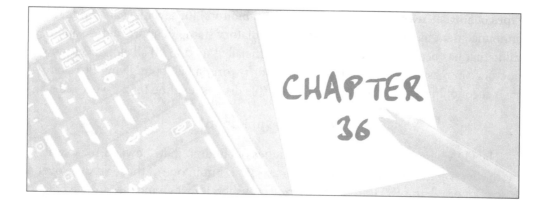

The P word:
FDA approves the use of Prozac for children

First ran 1/6/2003

Prozac for kids.

It sounds absurd, almost like a joke—like Viagra for kids, or HRT for kids. But I wasn't laughing last Friday when I turned on the evening news to hear that the FDA had approved Prozac for the treatment of depression and obsessive compulsive disorder in children aged 7 to 17.

They must have broken out the good champagne over at Eli Lilly & Company (maker of Prozac) to toast the expansion of an already lucrative market. But the sad fact is that hundreds of thousands of kids have already been taking Prozac (and other types of SSRIs—selective serotonin reuptake inhibitors) for several years. Friday's announcement by the FDA simply gives a regulatory stamp of approval for something that has been available (although not officially sanctioned) all along. But now doctors can reassure parents that they shouldn't worry a bit about giving Prozac to their second grader—because the FDA says this drug is just fine for a 7-year-old.

Into the unknown

The FDA based its approval on two studies of children that showed Prozac was more effective than placebo in fighting depression. But in one of those studies, over a 19-week period, the children taking Prozac grew about half an inch less (on average) than the children taking placebo. The children in the placebo group also gained an average of two pounds more than kids in the Prozac group. Regarding this, the FDA said, "The clinical significance of this observation on long-term growth is unknown."

As stamps of approval go, I find that one less than comforting. And it begs the question: If Prozac inhibits growth and weight gain, what is it doing to young brains as they grow and develop? No one knows the answer to that one.

What the studies DO show is that the side effects of Prozac are the same for children as they are for adults—including; dizziness, nausea, nervousness and difficulty concentrating. Of course, those last two are no problem. The pediatrician could always just write out a prescription for Ritalin to go along with the Prozac.

Sound absurd? What scares me is that it's probably already going on.

A better first option

According to Dr. Donald L. Rosenblitt, the medical director of the Lucy Daniels Center for Early Childhood, it's not unusual for physicians to prescribe Prozac, Zoloft or Paxil for children as young as 4 years old. As deplorable as that is, the real shame is that, beyond whatever environmental, social or personal circumstances might trigger depression, there are dietary factors that can and should be addressed long before any pediatrician offers the free "starter pack" of Prozac.

In an e-Alert I sent you last fall ("Omega Delta Blues" 10/28/02), I told you how those who experience mild to moderate depression often find relief with an increased intake of omega-3 fatty acids (in fish or fish oil supplements). People who are depressed are often deficient in magnesium, as well, which is found in whole grains, nuts and leafy green vegetables. Herbal supplements like valerian root, chamomile, black cohosh, and rosemary may also help manage depression. And the standout among the herbs for mild to moderate depression is, of course, St. John's wort, which is sometimes called the "natural Prozac" for its apparent ability to help manage the proper functioning of seratonin in the brain.

High levels of B vitamins have also been shown to relieve symptoms of depression. In addition to supplements, good dietary sources of vitamin B are: tuna, salmon, avocados, bananas, mangoes, potatoes, broccoli, cauliflower, poultry and meat. Note that stress (which often goes hand in hand with depression) is believed to deplete the body's store of B vitamins.

As pure as the Lilly white snow

In an Associated Press report last Friday, a spokesperson for Eli Lilly stated that the company "didn't intend to market Prozac for children." Right. I can't help but wonder if this spokesperson used to work for Phillip Morris. You and I both know that the FDA approval will have an absolute effect on the way Lilly's salespeople promote Prozac. With this new approval, doctors will feel more comfortable prescribing the drug for kids, and Lilly salespeople will certainly exploit the leverage of the FDA blessing.

If you're the parent or grandparent of a child who's struggling with depression, I urge you to explore the dietary and supplement options before you choose to medicate with a powerful drug whose long-term effects in children have not been adequately researched.

And if you have a friend or relative who is considering a pharmaceutical for their depressed child, I hope you'll forward this e-mail to them. Then when they're tempted by an easy answer and a "feel good" sales pitch (and they will be), they'll also know that they have another, less dangerous course of action to try first.

...and another thing

"An intake of more than 2,500 mcg of selenium per day, over a period of time, can be toxic."

This wasn't part of the dialogue from last week's "CSI: Crime Scene Investigation," but it could have been. That line was actually from an e-Alert I sent you last week ("Holiday Mix" 1/2/03) that discussed, among other things, the extremely remote chance that people can ingest a toxic amount of selenium—a naturally occurring mineral with powerful antioxidant properties.

We've talked about selenium many times before, of course. However, this time, the day after I sent that e-Alert, HSI Editorial Director Judy Douglas, e-mailed me to say: "CSI had two guys die of selenium poisoning last night—their wives did it, one with dandruff shampoo, the other with agricultural chemicals."

Hmmm...I wonder if the writers for CSI subscribe to the e-Alert. I guess we'll know for sure if an upcoming episode features a 7-year-old reacting to his Prozac.

To Your Good Health,

Jenny Thompson
Health Sciences Institute

Sources:

- "Prozac Cleared for Kids" Associated Press, 1/3/03
- "FDA Approves Prozac for Pediatric Population" Reuters Health, 1/3/03
- "Another Risk For Kids—Lots of Them On Prozac" Joyce Howard Price, The Washington Times, 9/7/98
- "U.S. Attention Deficit On Legal Drug Risks" Arianna Huffington, Arianna Online, 12/7/98

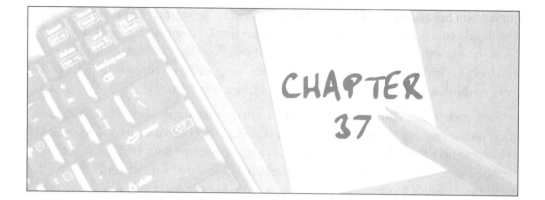

Consumer retort: Revealing the biased mainstream mindset

First ran 1/8/2003

Well, it came. Right there, amid the holiday bills and what seemed like hundreds of catalogs announcing after-Christmas sales, was my latest issue of Consumer Reports.

And they're at it again. This morning, when I saw the first article in the February issue of Consumer Reports, I was so frustrated that I immediately sat down to tell you about it. (I should really just read CR at my computer.) Because, once again, their "information" is no more than a completely biased view, based on a mainstream mindset.

Hot potato

The article in question calls for a ban on the herb, ephedra (also known as ma huang), which has received a lot of negative press in recent years for its potentially dangerous side effects. In general, HSI has shied away from recommending ephedra, because, although it can be a useful supplement (employed in Chinese medicine for hundreds of years), we also recognize its dangers—especially for those with heart problems, or those who don't follow recommended dosage instructions.

Ephedra contains ephedrine alkaloids that can have an amphetamine-like stimulant effect on the nervous system and heart. Historically, it has been used as one ingredient in multiple herb formulas—most designed to treat respiratory ailments. Problems occurred when the ephedrine content of the herb was isolated and concentrated. As it began to be included in more weight loss products, as a stimulant and appetite suppressant, people began using more than the recommended dosages. Following reports of seizures, heart attacks and even death, many companies pulled products containing ephedra from their shelves, and the AMA called for a complete ban of the herb.

As you would expect, Consumer Reports sides with the AMA and the mainstream consensus that if an herbal supplement can kill people, then it should be struck completely from the marketplace.

Seeing what they want to see

According to the FDA, about 14,000 unintentional overdoses of this product result in about 100 deaths each year. But this isn't an ephedra statistic. This statistic concerns a product that can be found on shelves in every grocery store and in just about any medicine cabinet in the U.S.—acetaminophen. That's right: Tylenol, and literally hundreds of other over-the-counter products that contain acetaminophen. But 100 deaths per year is probably a low estimate, because many hospitals don't report unintentional poisonings.

How many people have died as a result of taking ephedra? A search on the web brings conflicting numbers, but the highest estimate I could find was 81. That's not 81 per year—that's 81 over a period of eight years.

Meanwhile, on the Consumer Reports web site I searched for articles about acetaminophen. I found seven. One article mentions a woman who received multiple doses of acetaminophen from various sources, resulting in liver toxicity from which she quickly recovered. None of the other six articles addresses any side effects of the drug. And none of the seven articles reveal that scores of people die each year from acetaminophen overdose.

And I expect you won't be surprised to learn that Consumer Reports has not called for a complete ban of acetaminophen.

Balance

Without question, ephedra is a potent botanical that should be used with caution. And I agree that the public should be educated about the dangers of the herb. But I don't think that state and local laws need to be passed to protect people from ephedra (one of CR's recommendations), and I believe that calling for a ban of the supplement is an overreaction.

Without any laws being passed, and without any FDA directives, guidelines for ephedra dosage and label warnings were drafted in 1994 by the American Herbal Products Association, in collaboration with the National Nutritional Food Association and the Utah Natural Products Association. The draft was revised and adopted in 2000 by the Consumer Health Products Association.

Herbal product manufacturers have recognized the dangers of ephedra and their responsible reaction has been in the best interest of the public. Consumer Reports would serve their readers far better by acknowledging this and putting their efforts toward a balanced reporting of the dangers of ephedra rather than an over-the-top campaign to have ephedra banned.

As I've said a number of times before: Consumer Reports should stick to what it does best: rating toasters, microwave ovens and cell phones. Their writing about serious health care is akin to TV Guide telling me what stocks to buy. It's simply not their job.

...and another thing

Over the holidays I sent you e-Alerts about the pleasures and health benefits of two beverages: African Red Bush Tea ("Baltimore Tea Party" 12/26/02) and a white wine—Paradoxe Blanc—especially developed to contain as much of the antioxidant polyphenol as red wines ("Bob's Your Uncle" 12/31/02).

HSI member responses to both e-Alerts have been mostly along the lines of: "Where can I get some?"

A member named Lynn wrote: "I went to Baltimore Coffee and Tea online to order African red bush tea. They could not locate it for me. Please, can you give me any further information as to where I can order this tea?"

The African Red Bush Tea (which I'm still enjoying quite a bit) can be ordered from the Baltimore Coffee and Tea Company by phone (800-823-1408), or you can go to their web site (baltcoffee.com). This site is huge and takes some doing to navigate. Click on "Our Famous Tea Collection"—then click on "Eastern Shore Tea Company Loose Teas—Unique blends & flavors..." When that page comes up you'll see more than 50 teas listed in alphabetical order. Scroll down until you find "Eastern Shore Red Bush (Rooibos) Tea."

As I said, it will take a little doing to find it, but that's a snap compared to finding Paradoxe Blanc.

HSI member Andrea sent this e-mail: "OK, already, you've got me intrigued! Where can I BUY some of this Paradoxe Blanc wine?"

While researching the wine e-Alert, I came across several reports that claim the wine is now commercially available, but with zero information about where to find it. After checking at my local wine store, and searching several wine web sites on the Internet (one of which boasted having more than 2,500 different wines for sale), I'm beginning to suspect that Paradoxe Blanc may only be available in France right now.

If there are any dedicated wine connoisseurs out there who know where and how we might come by a bottle of PB, please write and let us know!

To Your Good Health,

Jenny Thompson

Health Sciences Institute

Sources:

- "Working To Get Ephedra Banned" Consumer Reports, February, 2003
- "Ephedra: Guidelines For Dosage And Label Warnings" SupplementQuality.com, October 2000
- "Ephedra Facts" The Ephedra Education Council
- "Over-The-Counter Drugs: How Safe?" Consumer Reports
- "Petition Filed to Ban Ephedra Supplements" Nutrition News Focus
- "Toxicity, Acetaminophen" Susan E. Farrell, M.D., Emedicine.com
- "Clearer Liver Warning Urged for Painkillers" Adam Marcus, Health Scout News, 9/20/02

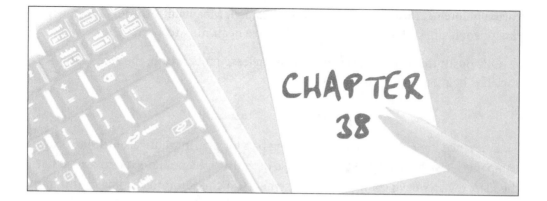

Muzzle on the watchdog: FDA's role in reviewing pharmaceutical company advertising

First ran 1/13/2003

Imagine a Snake Oil salesman rolls into town and gives a pitch that claims his product will rejuvenate the weary with no side effects. But the local sheriff knows that Snake Oil makes only one in five folks feel slightly less sluggish, and usually causes swelling of the feet. The sheriff asks the town's attorney to draw up an order to require the salesman to stop making his misleading claims. In the meantime he allows the salesman to continue his sales pitch.

A few days later, when the legal order is ready, the salesman is long gone, having sold his product to townspeople who know and trust that the sheriff always carefully reviews the claims of traveling salesmen. Meanwhile, throughout town, most people are still feeling weary and feet are beginning to swell.

Obviously, this is flawed system. Nevertheless, in our world, the role of the sheriff is being played by the FDA.

Something's burning

Ever since the FDA lifted an advertising ban for pharmaceuticals in 1996, drug companies have been allowed to advertise directly to the public. One caveat is that the FDA reviews drug company advertisements to check for misleading claims and to verify the inclusion of required warnings. But the loophole, (and since we're dealing with drug companies, you knew there had to be one) is that ads are allowed to run while they are still under review. Not only does this make the review process somewhat pointless, but potentially dangerous for consumers, as well.

Here's a perfect example.

Protopic is an ointment that treats eczema. The television ad for Protopic claimed that it "Soothes eczema anywhere on your body." The FDA ordered Protopic maker Fujisawa Healthcare to pull the ad, citing studies that showed how 25% of Protopic users experience itching, and almost half develop a burning sensation. So Fujisawa stopped running the ad, but by then who knows how many eczema patients had started to feel the burn?

Who needs muscles anyway?

Here's another good one.

A print ad for Lipitor stated that other cholesterol-lowering drugs cause "serious muscle damage." The implication, of course, was that Lipitor does not cause muscle damage. But in fact ALL statin drugs have the potential to cause muscle damage, including Lipitor. So during the weeks the FDA was busy preparing a legal review of its cease and desist letter (which it's required to do by the Department of Health and Human Services), Pfizer (the maker of Lipitor) was free to run the ad. Meanwhile, almost certainly, a number of statin drug users asked their doctors to switch their medication to Lipitor, believing they were avoiding muscle damage.

Regulation 101

Now, admittedly, this is a bit of a gray area for me. I certainly believe in less regulation, not more. But if we're going to have it and we're going to pay for it (I'm sure the FDA review isn't cheap), make it mean something.

Just these couple of examples demonstrate how ineffective this regulatory process is. Nevertheless, many in the mainstream medical establishment continue to call for the regulation of supplement manufacturers, as if the FDA has a reliable track record of sorting out the genuine from the false and putting effective controls in place.

In an e-Alert I sent you last week ("The P Word" 1/6/03), we saw the FDA in typical form, giving approval to prescribe Prozac to kids as young as seven, while admitting that the long term effects of Prozac on developing brains is unknown— as if to say, "Oh, don't worry about that. How bad could it be?" This is the sort of arbitrary protection you get from lumbering bureaucracies: half-baked, at best.

Meanwhile, in another recent e-Alert ("Consumer Retort" 1/8/03), I told you how herbal product manufacturers responded when the dangers of the botanical ephedra became known. They regulated themselves. Without any laws being passed, and without any FDA directives, strict guidelines for ephedra dosage and label warnings were drafted by three different herbal product associations, and adopted by the Consumer Health Products Association.

Home made

Whether you and I look to the FDA as a source of protection or not, a vast majority of Americans do. So they believe that when a pharmaceutical company makes a claim in an advertisement, that claim has been screened for accuracy. Based on that expectation, people are making personal health care decisions. Drug companies (fully aware of the weaknesses of this process) take advantage of the situation to spread misinformation about their products. In many cases, by the time an FDA order to pull an offending advertisement is received, the ads have already had their run and are no longer being aired or printed. By then consumers are already making choices based on misinformation.

This situation underlines the need for all health care consumers to understand the holes in the process and to ask questions and do their own research about any drug or supplement before beginning or changing a regimen. As always, the most reliable regulation starts at home.

To Your Good Health,

Jenny Thompson
Health Sciences Institute

Sources:

- "Free Rein For Drug Ads?" Consumer Reports, February, 2003
- "Prescription Drug Costs Back on Lawmakers' Agenda" Ellyn Ferguson, Gannett News Service, 5/15/02

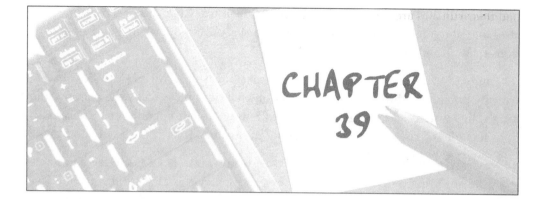

Annual tradition: Drug companies seek to expand the market for their existing products

First ran 1/29/2003

In an e-Alert dated exactly one year ago today ("More Bad News About Remicade and Enbrel" 1/29/02), I gave you the latest information on the disturbing side effects of two prescription drugs used to treat rheumatoid arthritis (RA) and Crohn's disease. Back then I said, "Unfortunately, the news gets even worse," and told you about research that showed both drugs may cause nerve damage that can lead to MS and other central nervous system disorders.

A year later, unfortunately, the news continues to get even worse.

Adding to the list

Earlier this month Reuters Health reported that two large clinical trials evaluating Enbrel in the treatment of congestive heart failure (CHF) had been stopped after one of the trials revealed that Enbrel was suspected of causing CHF conditions to WORSEN in patients.

Enbrel (the brand name for etenercept) was approved by the FDA in 1998 to treat rheumatoid arthritis. Taken by injection (self-administered by the patient), the drug's label warns that "allergic reactions to Enbrel are not uncommon." These reactions include the risk of infections, swelling in the deep layers of the skin, and hives.

Now you might wonder why a drug, already known to have side effects ranging from the annoying to the severe, would be given two large trials, to test it for an indication it wasn't even intended for. The simple answer: money. And lots of it. A month's round of Enbrel doses costs each patient a staggering $1,500. No surprise then that sales of Enbrel grossed $907 million in 2001—an increase of nearly 18 percent over the previous year. So, again, no surprise that the manufacturers of Enbrel (a company named Immunex, in partnership with Wyeth), would make every attempt to expand the market for their bread-winner, in spite of the fact that the list of unpleasant side effects seems to grow as fast as the yearly revenue.

Loopholes & scams

And this is where Remicade comes in. Remicade (manufactured by Centocor, a subsidiary of Johnson & Johnson) is Enbrel's chief competitor. They were both approved by the FDA in 1998 to treat rheumatoid arthritis, they are both used to treat Crohn's disease (even though neither drug is approved for that), they have both been associated with disorders of the central nervous system (MS and Guillain-Barre syndrome), and now Enbrel joins Remicade in being known to worsen CHF symptoms.

Remicade, however, has one huge advantage over Enbrel: Remicade has to be administered intravenously in a doctor's office. Ironically, this apparent drawback has turned into a plus, because Medicare reimburses doctors 95 percent of the "average wholesale price" for drugs that have to be administered by a doctor. So in spite of the inconvenience, Medicare recipients receive a huge break on the exorbitant price. But guess what? Centocor reps are now being investigated for possible fraud in exploiting this system.

Some drug companies have boosted the Medicare reimbursements to physicians by inflating the average prices they report to the government. According to The New York Times, early last year Centocor posted a notice for physicians on its web site, detailing the "estimated revenue per patient" that doctors would reap by prescribing Remicade. It's easy to imagine how this sort of incentive might encourage a doctor to prescribe Remicade, before trying a low-cost generic drug called Methotrexate, which is also a standard treatment for rheumatoid arthritis.

Add to that the fact that Medicare paid out more than $140 million for Remicade in 2001 (almost a 300 percent jump over the amount paid out in 2000), and you don't have to wonder why Centocor has drawn a federal investigation.

There's GOT to be a better way—and there is

Whew! That's a mighty tangled web of over-priced medications, dangerous side effects, and dubious drug company maneuvers. The good news is that the whole mess is avoidable for many who may find far less expensive relief from RA and Crohns's disease with two natural alternatives.

At HSI, we've written extensively about therapies for both RA and Crohn's disease. In the February 2001 Members Alert newsletter, we told you about an oral supplement from Germany called Wobenzyme, a blend of pancreatic enzymes that clears the body of the excess antibodies that characterize an autoimmune disease. Studies have shown that Wobenzyme can prevent RA flare-ups and help lower levels of these antibodies, called circulating immune complexes.

And in October 2000, we wrote about the therapeutic yeast saccharomyces boulardii (SB), which nourishes and protects the healthy intestinal flora. At least two clinical studies have shown that SB can significantly reduce Crohn's symptoms compared to placebo.

If you or someone you care about has been prescribed Enbrel, Remicade, or even the lower-priced generic Methotrexate to treat RA or Crohn's disease, ask your health care provider about the natural alternatives before signing on for involved pharmaceutical procedures and their growing list of side effects.

...and another thing

Last week I bought a new portable compact disc player—the kind that plays

CDs like a Walkman. While getting familiar with how it works, I came across this notice printed on the back of the unit: "This compact disc player meets all safety standards and regulations of the FCC, DHHS and FDA."

Huh? Why on earth would the Food and Drug Administration have regulations about a CD player?

In the past I've given Consumer Reports magazine a hard time for dispensing half-baked advice on health care instead of doing what they're supposed to do: test and rate cars, kitchen appliances, and electronic devices like...well, like compact disc players! And now the FDA has regs for CD players!? Has the whole world gone mad!?

This is as pure a case of over-regulation as you're likely to find. You would think that meeting all safety standards and regulations of the Federal Communications Commission and the Department of Health and Human Services would be more than enough. But no—they have to drag in the FDA as well?

After enjoying a little rant about this at home (I gave my husband an earful) I settled down and did some research and found that apparently the FDA's role here has something to do with "radiation performance."

Hmmm. I wonder—would the radiation performance of a compact disc player come under the heading of "food" or "drug"?

To Your Good Health,

Jenny Thompson
Health Sciences Institute

Sources:

- "Enbrel Arthritis Drug May Worsen Heart Failure" Richard Woodman, Reuters Health, 1/8/03

- "Arthritis Drug May Worsen Congestive Heart Failure" Dr. Joseph Mercola, Mercola.com

- "Methods Used for Marketing Arthritis Drug Are Under Fire" Melody Petersen, The New York Times, 4/11/02

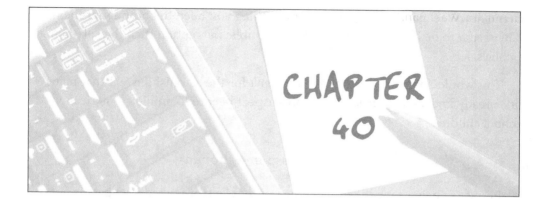

Don't beam me up: Irradiated beef

First ran 2/4/2003

If it walks like a duck, and it quacks like a duck, it's probably a duck. But then, you could always apply to the FDA to have the name "duck" changed to something more palatable, like "appealing fowl."

Last year the FDA announced that U.S. food companies planning to market irradiated beef may petition the agency to request the use of "neutral language" to describe their meat—something like "cold-pasteurized" rather than "irradiated"—a process that uses gamma rays or electrons to kill bacteria that cause food poisoning.

The fact that advocates of meat irradiation want to hide this process behind a brand new "feel good" name tells you everything you need to know about them: They seem to be far more concerned about public perception than they are about public safety.

This would be simply irritating if it weren't for the astonishing fact that plans are already underway to feed this highly suspect beef to 27 million American school children.

Warning signs ignored

In spite of being zapped with gamma rays or electrons, irradiated beef is not radioactive. And apparently the process is effective in killing bacteria like E. coli 0157:H7 and salmonella, both of which cause food poisoning. So what's the problem? Two things.

One: Studies in Europe have shown that irradiation may form cancer-causing agents in meat fat. The European Union has suspended the irradiation of beef and other foods (except for certain spices and herbs) until further studies have been completed.

Two: In a New York Times report last week, Carol Tucker Foreman (the director of the Food Policy Institute at the Consumer Federation of America) underlined the uncertain health risks of irradiation, saying, "There is nowhere in the world where a large population has eaten large amounts of irradiated food over a long period of time."

In short: We have good reason to suspect that irradiated meat may add up to serious health problems in the long run. But rather than rigorously test the process and make sure it's absolutely safe, Congress enacted a law last May directing the U.S. Department of Agriculture to allow irradiation of beef purchased for the federal school lunch program—a program that offers free or inexpensive meals to 27 million kids every school day.

If you go to the grocery store and see a package of meat that is clearly labeled "irradiated," or "cold pasteurized," or "never mind what we do to it—just trust us," you have a choice. You can choose non-irradiated meat, or fish, or vegetables. But a child standing in a lunch line is not exactly a discriminating consumer. He's far more likely to quickly eat what's put on his plate and make a mad dash for the playground, never giving the slightest thought about how the meat has been processed.

More than bargained for

The whole point of irradiation is to create a shortcut. When beef has been irradiated, there's no need to test for bacterial contamination. This is a time and money saving bonus for meat companies. But critics of the plan fear that this new system will encourage meat processors to cut corners on safety where they never dared before, creating relaxed sanitation standards that could considerably compromise meat quality.

But what about nutrition? This would seem to be an obvious question, but in the several articles I've read about irradiated beef, the subject of nutrition doesn't come up at all. So I asked HSI Panelist Allan Spreen, M.D., for his take on the way irradiation might affect nutrition, and he sent me this comment:

"Any electromagnetic radiation strong enough to kill undesirable elements in food is easily strong enough to do the same thing to desirable elements. Denaturing of enzymes, destruction of desirable bacteria, elimination of vital nutrients are all events that will be proven to occur once we get someone to study them. Since nobody has yet, why are 'we' so fired up about using the unproven technique on kids? (Wouldn't have anything to do with revenue enhancement for the food industry, would it?) The whole thing strikes me as unwholesome, and at the very least extremely premature."

Dodging gamma rays

Obviously, anyone who doesn't like the idea of irradiated beef can avoid it at the supermarket (trusting, of course, that it's clearly labeled). Beef dishes ordered in restaurants present another problem. But there is something you can do if you have children or grandchildren who benefit from the federal school lunch program.

The distribution of irradiated beef to schools may start as early as the 2003-2004 school year. At that time, school districts will have the right to refuse irradiated meat. Check with your school administrators to find out if they plan to serve irradiated beef. Tell them about your concerns and encourage them to postpone a decision to use this process until substantial further testing has been done. This is also a perfect time to get the word out to other parents at PTA meetings. Let them know about the potential dangers that irradiated meat poses to the children in your community.

The federal school lunch program benefits the children of low-income households. In many cases, these kids have no other source for their lunch meal. In other words, turning down the meal is not an option. All children deserve a nutritious school lunch, but they also deserve a safer solution to ensuring meat safety.

When I was in grade school, we had a name for cafeteria meat dishes like Sloppy Joe sandwiches and chipped beef: we called it mystery meat. Little did we know back then just how genuinely mysterious meat might someday become.

...and another thing

Speaking of mystery meat, last week a federal judge dismissed a lawsuit filed against McDonald's on behalf of children who claimed the fast food chain was responsible for making them obese.

As it turned out, the plaintiffs' suit didn't have much beef.

The judge ruled that plaintiffs failed to demonstrate that deceptive advertising was used by McDonald's, failed to show that McDonald's alone was responsible for their obesity, and failed to state the frequency that plaintiffs ate at McDonald's.

In his written opinion, U.S. District Court Judge Robert Sweet emphasized the personal responsibility of the plaintiffs, stating that it was not the court's place to protect them from their own poor judgment, "if they...choose to satiate their appetite with a surfeit of supersized McDonald's products."

In an e-Alert I sent you last summer ("Rendering Unto Caesar" 8/5/02) I told you about other lawsuits filed against McDonald's in which the plaintiffs placed full blame for their health problems on Big Macs—as if Big Macs and French fries had been forced on them. So I completely agree with Judge Sweet's view of personal responsibility.

But don't jump to the conclusion that this ruling might put the brakes on lawsuits aimed at McDonald's and other fast food franchises. Judge Sweet closed his opinion with the suggestion that an amended complaint could be filed, based on the probability that the plaintiffs had no way of knowing the dangers in certain menu items that are so completely processed they no longer resemble the food sources they came from. As an example, the judge singled out Chicken McNuggets, calling them a "McFrankenstein creation of various elements not utilized by the home cook."

I don't really agree with Judge Sweet on this point. I think that anyone who's eaten even a single McNugget (and believe me, I'm not recommending it) has all the evidence they need that it bears only the slightest possible resemblance to real food.

But I do think "McFrankenstein" is a nice touch. I'd love to know how the spin doctors at McDonald's corporate headquarters are handling that one.

To Your Good Health,

Jenny Thompson
Health Sciences Institute

Sources:

- "The Question of Irradiated Beef in Lunchrooms" Marian Burros, The New York Times, 1/29/03

- "Parents Protest U.S. Schools Irradiated Meat Plan" Randy Fabi, Reuters, 12/13/02

- "FDA Allowing Food Companies To Change Irradiation Label to 'Cold Pasteurization'" Reuters, 10/9/02

- "Obesity Suit Against McDonald's Dismissed" Consumer Health Digest #03-04, 1/28/03

- "Judge Tosses Out McDonald's Complaint, But Suggests Re-filing Under Novel Theory" Obesity Policy Report, 1/28/03

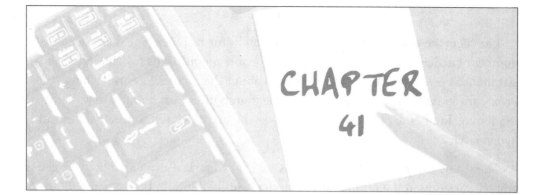

The under-over: Prescribing stimulant drugs for our kids

First ran 2/6/2003

I enjoy occasionally listening to National Public Radio, but sometimes I would swear the "P" in NPR stands for Pharmaceutical.

Monday morning, on my way in to work, I was listening to NPR when I heard a comment that nearly made me drive off the road. It wasn't exactly road rage— nothing that extreme—more like road shock. I'm not certain, but there's a good chance I shouted "I CAN'T BELIEVE MY EARS!" out loud.

Coast to coast

Life seems to deliver things in clusters. Lately, for instance, I've come across a number of articles and studies about questionable medications for children (see last month's e-Alert ("The P Word" 1/6/03) about the increase in prescribing Prozac for kids). So I wasn't surprised to hear an NPR report about a new study examining another aspect of the debate over the use of Ritalin to treat adolescent hyperactivity.

The study, reported in the February issue of "Pediatrics," evaluated the U.S. geographic variation in the number of children prescribed Ritalin throughout 1999. Approximately 178,000 cases were assessed, with children ranging in age from 4-15 years old. Two striking statistics stood out in the data. Allowing for variables such as regional population, researchers found that Ritalin use tends to be greater among kids in the Eastern U.S., as opposed to kids in the West. More specifically, the highest Ritalin use was in Louisiana (with more than 6 kids in 100 taking Ritalin), and the lowest was in Washington, D.C. (with 1.6 kids in 100 taking the drug).

Now there are all sorts of reasons why this wide disparity might exist. And I think the very fact that it DOES exist points up the arbitrary factors involved in diagnosing these so-called "disorders" of ADD (attention deficit disorder) and ADHD (attention deficit/hyperactivity disorder). But while addressing these regional differences in the data, NPR reporter Jackie Norton spoke the line that made me nearly leap through the sun-roof of my car: "The study doesn't address if the stimulant drugs are being underused in one area, or overused in another."

UNDERUSED! As if it's even remotely possible to under-prescribe stimulant drugs for children! As if there are poor, unfortunate kids out there who are being deprived of their daily dose of Ritalin!

Enough with the stimulation!

There is no such thing as a Ritalin deficiency. But there are hyperactive kids. And in almost every case the cause is dietary, and the solution is dietary change. These important points were made by HSI Panelist Allan Spreen, M.D., in an e-Alert I sent you last spring ("How To Dismantle an '89 Ford" 6/3/02). In that e-

Alert Dr. Speen pointed out that sensitivities to specific foods (or food additives, like dyes) can trigger hyperactivity. He also gave useful tips on how to go about discovering which foods are the culprits.

In addition, Dr. Spreen recommended various supplements that have been shown to help calm hyperactivity, such as; omega-3 fatty acids, vitamin E, magnesium (in doses not high enough to loosen stools), alpha lipoic acid, amino acid supplements like GABA and L-tryptophan, vitamin C in high doses, and finally, a good basic multi-vitamin/mineral regimen.

I know that the hectic pace of life that comes with raising kids makes the concept of dietary change much easier said than done. So believe me, I'm not passing any judgment on parents who opt for Ritalin, especially when they're often pressured to take the pharmaceutical route by pediatricians, school administrators and fed-up teachers.

The point is this: There are options to Ritalin. And anytime someone suggests that stimulant drugs like Ritalin might be "underused," they'll hear my over-stimulated cry of disbelief all the way from Louisiana to Washington, D.C.

...and another thing

As a sidebar to yesterday's e-Alert ("Over the Teeth, Past the Gums..." 2/5/03) about the association between periodontal disease and heart disease (and how antioxidants may be a significant supplementary treatment for both), I wanted to give you some additional dental information from another e-Alert I sent you some time ago ("HSI Panelist Shares Even More Risks From Antidepressants" 11/9/01).

The HSI Panelist mentioned in the title is HSI Panelist Richard Cohan, D.D.S., M.S., M.B.A., who offered a warning about a common side effect of pharmaceutical antidepressants. Xerostomia is the medical name for dryness of the mouth, which is caused by a dysfunction of the salivary glands.

Dr. Cohan wrote: "As a group, antidepressants cause more xerostomia than any other. And, as you may know, xerostomia leads to an increase in caries (cavities), periodontal disease, and candidiasis, a yeast infection in the mouth often referred to as thrush. While not everyone who takes antidepressants experiences these side effects, those who do are often left with serious, permanent damage. For instance, these conditions can lead to irreversible loss of periodontal support of the teeth and the loss of teeth themselves. Just more of the hidden dangers in taking these drugs."

And as we now know, to that list we can add, "increased risk of heart disease."

To Your Good Health,

Jenny Thompson
Health Sciences Institute

Sources:

- Ritalin Study Report, Jackie Norton, NPR Morning Edition, 2/3/03

- "Geographic Variation in the Prevalence of Stimulant Medication Use Among Children 5 to 14 Years Old: Results From a Commercially Insured US Sample" Pediatrics, Vol. 111 No. 2 February 2003, pp. 237-243

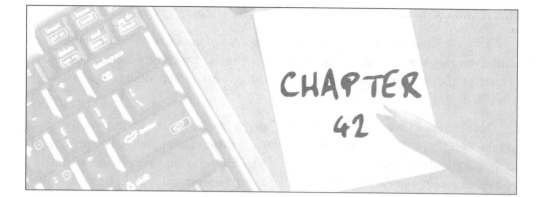

Ban the torpedoes: The real story behind Ephedra's fall from grace

First ran 3/3/2003

Since the tragic death two weeks ago of Steve Bechler, the young Baltimore Orioles pitcher who died of complications due to a history of heart problems presumably compounded by an intake of a diet supplement containing ephedrine, a firestorm of controversy has erupted.

The knee-jerk reaction from the medical mainstream has been predictable: a call for the ban of ephedra, demands for more explicit warning labels on ephedra bottles, and a general resumption of the discussion about treating herbal and dietary supplements as pharmaceuticals with all the attendant regulations.

What's under the hood?

This past Friday the FDA proposed that bottles of ephedra should be labeled with a warning that the herb may cause heart attack, stroke and death. FDA representatives also said that a ban on some ephedra-containing products is also being discussed.

This reference to "ephedra-containing" products is as close as they get to making the important distinction between two very different supplements: ephedra (an herb that should be used with caution and provides excellent relief from asthma), and ephedrine (a typical ingredient of diet formulations that should be used with extreme caution because the active component of ephedra is boosted to dangerously high levels).

To compare ephedra and ephedrine as if they are one and the same is like comparing a '65 beetle Volkswagen with a Formula One race car. Sure, they're both automobiles, but one has a top speed of MAYBE 80 miles per hour, while the other can more than triple that speed. Put someone who's not careful behind the wheel of either of these cars, and you'll get drastically different results.

But in the current public debate over the safety of ephedra and ephedrine, the two tend to be regarded as more or less one and the same. So they're usually referred to generically as "ephedra." As a result, the less dangerous herbal form of ephedra is getting the blame for the sins of ephedrine.

Risk assessment

In response to Friday's FDA announcement, Health and Human Services Secretary Tommy Thompson said, "Throughout America, there continue to be tragic incidents that link dietary supplements containing ephedra to serious health problems. I don't now why anyone would take these products. Why take the risk?"

I can't help but wonder if Secretary Thompson has ever taken an acetaminophen product such as Tylenol. A total of about 100 deaths have been attributed to complications involving "ephedra-containing" products. Meanwhile, the FDA estimates that the thousands of acetaminophen overdoses each year result in about 100 deaths. That's 100 PER YEAR!

But do we hear the FDA calling for a ban on acetaminophen? Of course not.

And don't even get me started on the risks associated with every prescription filled in this country every day.

If Secretary Thompson is puzzled about why people continue to take ephedra, do you suppose he also shakes his head and says, "I don't know why anyone would take prescription drugs or acetaminophen. Why take the risk?"

Keep in mind that this is the same man ready to line us all up and inject us with smallpox vaccines, knowing that hundreds or even thousands of Americans may suffer permanent debilitating side effects and death.

Self regulating

An Associated Press report about the FDA comments last Friday included this statement: "Because ephedra is an herb, U.S. law lets manufacturers sell it over-the-counter with little oversight to ensure safety."

Well...not exactly.

Ephedra is sold over-the-counter with little oversight from the FDA. That much is true. But the supplement industry has provided its own "oversight."

Without any laws being passed, and without any FDA directives, guidelines for ephedra dosage and label warnings were drafted in 1994 by the American Herbal Products Association, in collaboration with the National Nutritional Food Association and the Utah Natural Products Association. The draft was revised and adopted in 2000 by the Consumer Health Products Association.

Herbal product manufacturers have recognized the dangers of ephedra and their responsible reaction has been in the best interest of the public. An all-out ban of ephedra would only benefit pharmaceutical companies that sell asthma drugs.

And we will simply never be able to protect the people that choose to ignore warning labels or use products at dosages much higher than recommended.

...and another thing

I've told you about the benefits of eating berries in a number of past e-Alerts.

So even though this is old news for some of you, it never hurts to repeat it every now and then. Especially because many berries increase the levels of a flavonoid called quercetin—a highly effective antioxidant that has been shown to help provide protection against heart disease, lung cancer, asthma and type 2 diabetes.

A new study from the National Public Health Institute, Helsinki, Finland compared flavonoid levels in the blood of 40 men whose average age was 60. For eight weeks, half the group ate 100 grams a day of bilberries, blackcurrants, and lingonberries. The other 20 continued their normal diets.

Researchers found that men in the berry-eating group ingested more than twice the amount of quercetin than men in the non-berry group. Over a long period of time, this higher intake of quercetin could have a very positive effect on health, especially since berries are also rich in vitamin C and natural fiber. Bilberries are also believed to help prevent age related macular degeneration.

The Helsinki researchers noted that raw berries are preferable to berries that are frozen or cooked because freezing and heating can destroy some antioxidants.

To Your Good Health,

Jenny Thompson
Health Sciences Institute

Sources:

- "FDA Proposes Warning Labels for Ephedra" Lauran Neergaard, Associated Press, 2/28/03
- Berries: A Great Source of Plant Antioxidants" Dr. Joseph Mercola, mercola.com

Choose your poison: Seperating myth from fact in the Ephedra debate

First ran 3/6/2003

The current debate over the safety of ephedra is no longer a debate—it's turned into the sort of emotional, high-pitched squabbling that makes you want to blast a whistle and ask everyone to calm down, take a deep breath, stand back, and look at the realities behind the myths.

Because when you expose the myths behind this debate, it becomes almost no debate at all.

The infamous "100"

Believe me, what you're about to read, you won't find in your local newspaper, or on network TV. They're so busy putting up packaged sound bites from the medical mainstream (with all the familiar acronyms: FDA, HHS, AMA) that they don't have time to outline the finer points that contain the truth of the ephedra debate.

MYTH: More than 100 deaths have been attributed to ephedra usage.

FACT: The statistics on ephedra-related deaths don't hold up.

The FDA received more than 800 adverse event reports concerning ephedra between 1993 and 1997. Included in the reports: a man who was taking ephedra died of a gunshot wound; a woman who had been taking ephedra died in a car accident; a man who had been taking ephedra died of environmental hyperthermia; and so on. To say the least, it's quite a stretch to blame these untimely deaths on the completely incidental fact that the victims were using ephedra. I imagine all of those people were wearing shoes too, but I doubt anyone blamed shoes for their deaths.

In the current issue of HSI Panelist Jon Barron's Baseline of Health Newsletter, Jon writes, "The case against ephedra is based on statistical nonsense." Jon points out that in the studies examining groups of subjects who used ephedra products against groups of subjects who did not, there was no statistical difference in the rate of strokes or heart attacks.

Cascade of events

MYTH: Ephedra killed Baltimore Orioles pitcher Steve Bechler.

FACT: Several different factors led to Bechler's death. Ephedra was not one of them.

A bottle of Xenadrine RFA-1, a weight-loss supplement containing ephedrine (NOT ephedra, but a boosted component of the herb ephedra) was found in Bechler's locker. A teammate reported that Bechler had taken three capsules of Xenadrine on the morning of his death (not yet confirmed by the medical examiner's toxicology report which has yet to be completed). According to instructions on the Xenadrine label, three capsules are to be taken throughout the day, not all at once.

One week after his death, three doctors at the Baylor University Center for Exercise, Nutrition and Preventive Health Research released a special report listing the dangerous factors that contributed to Steve Bechler's death:

- A prior history of heart illness

- A family history of death due to heatstroke

- A history of liver problems and high blood pressure

- Bechler had reported to spring training camp several pounds overweight (and was highly motivated to lose the weight in order to win a spot in the Orioles pitching rotation)

- Bechler was wearing several layers of clothing during workouts in an apparent attempt to help his weight-loss regimen

- Bechler may have not yet been acclimatized to the heat and humidity of South Florida (spring training had just begun the week he died)

- Bechler had eaten no solid food for as much as two days before his death

- When Bechler collapsed on the field, his core temperature was 106 degrees

Dr. Joshua Perper, the Broward County (Fla.) Medical Examiner, stated that the Xenadrine label clearly states that those with heart problems, hypertension or liver problems should not take the supplement. So if Steve Bechler had followed the manufacturers guidelines, he would never have taken ephedrine at all.

If for some reason I choose to drink gasoline and I were to die from it, would the FDA ban the sale of gasoline? And should my family sue Exxon? No. Because I was using the product in a way it was not intended to be used. And that's exactly what happened here—and in the majority of other cases where ephedrine is seen as the "killer." Ephedrine is not intended to be used in these doses by people with certain health conditions.

Looking the other way

MYTH: The FDA bans food or drug products that are dangerous.

FACT: The arbitrary nature of FDA bans defies logic.

Aspartame is perhaps the most notoriously harmful food additive. Better known by its brand names—Equal and Nutra-sweet—aspartame has been shown to either mimic or worsen diseases such as Parkinson's, multiple sclerosis, Alzheimer's, arthritis, lupus, fibromyalgia, and depression. In short—it's FDA approved poison.

The FDA maintains an Adverse Reaction Monitoring System (ARMS) to track complaints about the unpleasant side effects of drugs, supplements and food additives. Reports of health problems resulting from an intake of aspartame make up approximately 75 percent of the total complaints received. In 1994 the Department of Health and Human Services (HHS) released a list of 61 reported adverse reactions to aspartame, including: chest pains, asthma, arthritis, migraine headaches, insomnia, seizures, tremors, vertigo, and weight gain.

So has either the FDA or HHS called for a ban of aspartame? No. Has either of the agencies even called for a warning label? No. In fact, the FDA has resisted efforts to establish a warning label for aspartame, stating (completely contrary to all the evidence) that the complaints against the sweetener aren't sufficient enough to warrant such a label!

And have you heard the media calling for us to immediately remove every (heavily advertised) diet soft drink from our grocery store shelves to protect the public from the awful risk? After all, we're supposed to drink that "just for the taste of it." So to quote HHS Secretary Tommy Thompson, "Why would anybody take the risk?"

Witch hunt mentality

The current ephedra situation reminds me of a similar controversy involving l-tryptophan, a dietary supplement, used as a natural alternative to pharmaceutical sleeping medications. In 1989 there was a sudden rash of serious allergic reactions to l-tryptophan that resulted in 38 deaths. The problem was tracked down to a manufacturing short cut taken by one Japanese producer that had introduced a contaminant they didn't know about. L-tryptophan had been used for years without difficulty. But all it took was one bad batch. The FDA banned supplements of l-tryptophan in 1990.

When herbal formulations or dietary supplements begin to be perceived as dangerous, the medical mainstream moves quickly to demonize them—and by association, they demonize the supplement industry. This time, the demonizing process is gaining momentum daily. Congressmen and other government representatives see what appears to be a no-brainer issue and rush to publicly condemn the killer ephedra, many of them apparently unaware that ephedra is a far cry from ephedrine. Even the liberal lobby organization Public Citizen has threatened to sue the FDA to force a ban on ephedra.

It's quite amazing to see Public Citizen demanding that the government intervene to block everyone's access to an effective and useful herb (that has probably saved many more lives than it is accused of ending) in order to protect a few people who choose not to use it properly.

Meanwhile, no one seems to notice that this process is steadily legislating ourselves away from the freedom to make our own healthcare choices. Let your representatives in Congress know how you feel about this issue by sending them an e-mail. You can easily find e-mail addresses for congressmen and other government officials at a web site called Congress.org. If you prefer to write the old-fashioned way, you can find the appropriate mailing addresses at the same site.

And I hope you'll share this information with your friends and family too. Let them know that the information they've been hearing about ephedra in the mainstream press is not only short on reality, it's also a threat to our right to choose.

...and another thing

Last week I sent you an e-Alert ("Breaking the Code" 2/24/03) about a new coding system for doctors called Advanced Billing Concept Codes (ABC Codes), that has the potential to completely change the way alternative healthcare is prescribed and covered by insurance. This could be a huge benefit to the patients of practitioners who are members of groups such as the American Association of Oriental Medicine, the World Chiropractic Alliance, the Midwives Alliance of North America, the Acupuncture and Oriental Medicine Alliance, the American Massage Therapy Association, and the American Nurses Association.

But there's a catch. The ABC pilot program requires registration in order to participate, and the deadline for registration is March 16, 2003. Anyone unregistered by that date will not be able to use the codes during the two-year trial period.

In the February e-Alert I suggested that you call your doctor (or your chiropractor, or your acupuncturist, etc.) to find out if he's registered in the pilot program. That comment prompted a question from an HSI member named Audrey who says she spoke to her doctors, "but they do not know where to get the forms to register for this pilot program. Can you help?"

Happy to help, Audrey. Healthcare practitioners, and organizations that would like to participate can register at this web site: www.alternativelink.com.

Registration is available only through the Alternative Link web site. But the deadline is drawing near, so don't delay. Call your healthcare provider immediately and urge him to participate in this groundbreaking program.

To Your Good Health,

Jenny Thompson
Health Sciences Institute

Sources:

■ "FDA Rolling Out Ephedra Warning Labels" Lauran Neergaard, Associated Press, 3/2/03

■ "Interesting Times" Jon Barron & Kristen Barron, Baseline of Health Newsletter, 3/3/03, jonbarron.com

■ "The History of the FDA's Opposition to Ephedra" Ephedra Education Council, ephedrafacts.com

■ "The Alleged Role of Ephedra in the Death of a Professional Baseball Player" Kreider, Greenwood & Greenwood, Exercise & Sport Nutrition Lab, Center for Exercise, Nutrition and Preventive Health Research, Baylor University, 2/21/03

■ "Reported Aspartame Toxicity Effects" Holistic Healing Web Page, holisticmed.com

■ "Aspartame...The BAD News!" Mark Gold, doorway.com

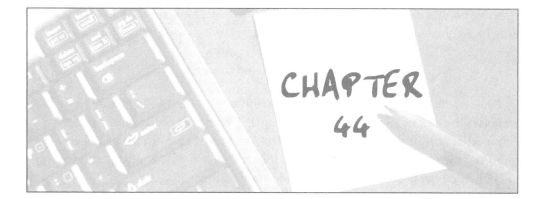

Spin this: More HRT risks revealed in major medical study

First ran 5/29/2003

It's hard enough to put a good spin on bad news, but when the news trend keeps going from bad to worse, all the spin in the world won't make a rotten egg fresh again.

Yesterday the Journal of the American Medical Association (JAMA) released more results from the Women's Health Initiative study on synthetic hormone replacement therapy (HRT). This time the medical mainstream was expecting good news about HRT and Alzheimer's disease. They were in for a shock.

As an e-Alert reader and HSI member you already know that there are safe and effective natural alternatives to prescription HRT. But now, more than ever, it's time to get the word out and tell your friends.

A fly in the ointment

By now you've probably heard the television news sound bites stating that HRT increases the risk of Alzheimer's. But as usual, TV talking heads rarely stop to define what constitutes this particular "HRT," and most of them haven't been reporting the full story that clearly underlines the fact that the most popular form of HRT (the type used in these studies) is simply dangerous.

Here's a quick recap of the new study: More than 4,500 women, aged 65 and older, were divided into two groups. Half took a placebo, and the other half took Prempro, an HRT combination of estrogen and progestin. Four years later, the women in the HRT group had developed Alzheimer's disease at TWICE the rate of those taking placebo (40 in the HRT group, and 21 in the placebo).

To say this was a surprise to researchers is to put it mildly. The exact opposite results had been hoped for.

Spin cycle

Right away the mainstream started spinning the news, pointing out that only a small number of women actually developed Alzheimer's. My personal favorite spin came from Dr. Samuel E. Gandy, vice chairman of the medical and scientific advisory council of the Alzheimer's Association, who told the New York Times that, "A small number doubled is still a small number."

I can't help but think that statement could only come from someone who's not taking the medication. What looks small to Dr. Gandy probably appears quite large to those women who can now thank synthetic HRT for sending them down the road toward Alzheimers. And I can't imagine most of these women are thinking, "Oh, that's just a small number, la de da."

Given the fact that there are already many doctors prescribing this particular HRT therapy to prevent Alzheimer's, Dr. Gandy's comment misses the point completely. Prempro doesn't prevent Alzheimer's at all—it increases the risk.

But that's only part of the problem. The current issue of JAMA also carries two additional reports. One found that women using HRT performed poorly on cognitive tests compared to women taking placebo, and the other confirmed earlier studies that demonstrated how Prempro increases the risk of stroke.

So here's the "logic" behind taking Prempro: Estrogen has been shown to cause cancer of the uterus. So Prempro combines estrogen with progestin, which protects the uterus. In other words, when you're taking Prempro, you're taking a medication that causes cancer, along with a "protective" agent that has now been shown to increase the risk of Alzheimer's, breast cancer, stroke, and gallstones.

What's wrong with this picture!?

Healthy voices

In an e-Alert I sent you last year ("Hiding The R" 11/4/02) I told you about a common trigger for menopausal side effects called "estrogen dominance," which is an imbalance between two hormones: estrogen and progesterone. Many women report remarkable results in maintaining hormonal balance with natural progesterone treatments (such as progesterone cream) that are available without a doctor's prescription.

Several HSI members shared the natural methods that have worked for them in a December e-Alert ("Turning Down The Heat" 2/17/02). Donna, for instance, wrote to tell about the effectiveness of a wild yam progesterone cream, "...a friend of mine told me she was using a cream called yam cream. Guess what? It worked great! I rarely had a hot flash from then on."

Jeanne told us that taking the element indium, as indium sulfate, "proved to be an absolute miracle" in reducing hot flashes and anxiety, while restoring energy and concentration. And a member named Glo said that daily doses of 2000 mg of vitamin C and 400 IU of vitamin E reduced her frequency of hot flashes from 10 each day, to only one.

We also heard from a Dr. V. who added this nutritional advice: "Please do not forget those wonderful [omega-3] essential fatty acids for hormonal health. I cannot tell you the degree of satisfaction I achieve just adding essential fatty acids, equivalent of 2-3 tbsp. daily, and digestive enzymes, preferably broad spectrum and above average potency, along with watching your starch or complex carb intake. Don't forget the importance also of eating fermented foods such as organic yogurt (no fat free stuff), sauerkraut, and apple cider vinegar. The health of your intestinal flora will also keep healthy estrogens recirculating thereby helping to control pre-ms and post-ms symptoms. We should always choose natural over synthetic hormones."

And I've also told you about various botanical treatments (most notably black cohosh and red clover) that have been shown to help maintain hormonal balance.

Share the news

With all the known dangers of synthetic combination HRT therapy, it's becoming harder to imagine why women would use this treatment without first trying alternatives that don't carry the risk of debilitating or life-threatening diseases.

Please share this e-Alert with friends and family members who might be using or considering the use of prescription drugs to address the concerns of menopause. Let them know they don't have to place their health at risk in return for comfort and peace of mind.

...and another thing

This past Monday things got ugly in Lancaster, England. It was almost as if a bull was turned loose in a china shop, but not quite.

On my way home from work yesterday I heard a report on National Public Radio about a bull that escaped from a cattle market in northeast England, then made a bee line into a nearby antiques store. Not quite a china shop, but it'll do.

Was the bull looking for refuge, or was it just in the mood for some mischief? We'll never know, but once inside the shop it did what any bull would do in the same situation. It ran amok. Terrified customers fled for the exits as gravy boats sailed through the air and grandfather clocks tipped like dominos. No doubt, some fine china was crunched under hoof.

And this story taught us what eventually must happen to a bull in a china shop, or an antiques shop, or probably any kind of shop: the police shot him. Not nice, perhaps, but where are you going to get a tranquilizer gun on short notice in Lancaster?

While writing today's e-Alert, I thought to compare synthetic HRT to a bull in a china shop. At some point the risks become too great to do nothing. Maybe it's time the medical police pull that trigger.

To Your Good Health,

Jenny Thompson
Health Sciences Institute

Sources:

- "Estrogen Plus Progestin and the Incidence of Dementia and Mild Cognitive Impairment in Postmenopausal Women" Journal of the American Medical Association, 2003;289:2651-2662, jama.ama-assn.org

- "Effect of Estrogen Plus Progestin on Global Cognitive Function in Postmenopausal Women" Journal of the American Medical Association, 2003;289: 2663-2672, jama.ama-assn.org

- "Hormone Use Found to Raise Dementia Risk" Denise Grady, The New York Times, 5/28/03, nytimes.com

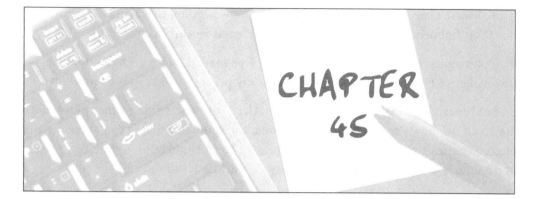

Working dark wonders: NY Times reveals shocking drug company maneuver

First ran 6/2/2003

A woman I know named Betty has been battling ovarian cancer for almost two years. Recently, a new round of chemotherapy really hit her hard so her doctor suggested they try Procrit to take the edge off the chemo side effects.

I'm sure you've probably seen the many Procrit commercials that have been running on national television for a few months now. The ads feature people who are fatigued because of chemo related anemia, but Procrit can also be prescribed for other health problems that cause anemia, such as kidney disease, HIV treatments, and recovery from surgery.

So I wasn't surprised when Betty told me she was going to start taking Procrit. But I was flabbergasted when she told me that each weekly dose will cost $1,000!

Outrageous? In my opinion, yes. But in a free market society, Ortho Biotech (the maker of Procrit) has the right to place any price tag it likes on its product.

But Procrit isn't the subject of today's e-Alert. It just so happens that Betty told me about her new Procrit regimen on almost the same day that I read about a pharmaceutical company atrocity that I believe has a connection to the high price of patent drugs. And calling it an "atrocity" is putting it mildly.

A bottom line plan

A recent investigative report conducted by the New York Times details one of the most despicable drug company maneuvers that I've ever heard.

Cutter Biological (a division of the German pharmaceutical giant Bayer) manufactures a blood-clotting agent for hemophiliacs. The product, called Factor VIII, contains human blood plasma. In the early 80s, AIDS presented a grave problem when it became apparent that Factor VIII and similar products made by other drug companies could easily spread the disease. A process was quickly developed that removed the threat of contaminating the drug with AIDS. But thousands of units of the unimproved and unsafe product had already been manufactured.

Without question, those unsafe units had to be dumped, right? A drug company is dedicated to providing products that improve their customers' health, right? No one with good conscience could possibly allow those contaminated units to be sold, right? And you know exactly where I'm going with this, right?

Cutter's solution: Sell the improved Factor VIII in America, and sell the unsafe product in Asia and South America. And not only did they sell the unsafe Factor VIII after they knew it would put hemophiliac patients in jeopardy, they continued to manufacture the contaminated product for another five months!

Quickly...quietly

Because of poor record keeping in the early years of the AIDS epidemic, it's impossible to know exactly how many hemophiliac patients contacted AIDS because of Cutter's bottom line business decision. What IS known is that a number of patients were infected and died while Cutter maintained its profit margin. A doctor in Taiwan reported that in one hemophiliac clinic alone, 44 patients developed AIDS. To date, 23 of them have died, including a 2-year-old.

Cutter has never admitted any wrongdoing in this matter, and Bayer has defended its subsidiary, stating that the company behaved "responsibly, ethically, and humanely." (So now we know what passes for responsible, ethical, and humane in the drug industry!)

But the FDA didn't agree. When FDA officials got wind of the matter in 1985, they summoned representatives of Cutter and the other companies that manufactured the product to explain that it was not acceptable to ship their contaminated medication overseas. One FDA administrator then asked that the problem be settled "quickly and quietly," adding that there was no reason to alert the public, the medical community, or Congress.

Ouch! That showed them! A gentle slap on the wrist for spreading a lethal disease.

If the lawsuit fits...

It's estimated that Cutter made more than $4 million dollars after allowing the sale of medication they knew was unsafe. So far, Bayer and the three other companies that sold this contaminated product have paid out almost $600 million to settle lawsuits.

And what does that have to do with the price of Procrit? Well, when drug companies solve problems by throwing money at them, someone has to pay. And that someone is the consumer.

Inevitably, whenever drug companies are challenged for charging exorbitant prices for drugs, they point to the high cost of research and development, without acknowledging that their legal departments spend millions (maybe billions) each year to make lawsuits disappear—lawsuits created by inadequately tested drugs or reckless business decisions.

So the next time you hear about a drug that costs more per dose than some used cars, you'll know that one of the things that consumers of that drug are almost certainly paying for is the price tag of making ugly situations go away "quickly and quietly."

The alternative

As a post script, I have some information about a natural way to address anemia that is considerably less expensive than Procrit.

In a Members Alert we sent you last spring (April 2002) we told you about a botanical called Energy Kampo. In Japan, this formulation of 10 herbal ingredients is called Juzen-taiho-to and is used for a wide variety of conditions. People struggling with chronic diseases (including rheumatoid arthritis, ulcerative colitis, atopic dermatitis, and chronic fatigue syndrome) take it to ease fatigue, anemia, circulatory problems, night sweats, and loss of appetite. Cancer patients take it to improve their overall condition and lessen the adverse effects of chemotherapy, radiation, and surgery.

If you're dealing with the effects of cancer treatments, or if you have a close friend or loved one who is coping with cancer related anemia, you can find out more information about Energy Kampo from a New York City nutritional pharmacy called Willner Chemists (willner.com/honso.htm).

...and another thing

Last week I heard from our friend William Campbell Douglas, M.D., the editor of Real Health Newsletter, who had some important insights on an e-Alert I sent you about the ineffectiveness of the pneumonia vaccine ("Revealing The Matrix" 5/21/03).

I told you about the results of a large study that showed how the pneumonia vaccination simply does not reduce the risk of pneumonia in older adults. Nevertheless, the researchers concluded by reasserting the recommendation that all seniors should receive the vaccine because their study indicated that it reduced the risk of contracting the relatively uncommon condition called pneumococcal bacteremia.

But even that flimsy basis for promoting the vaccine is insupportable, according to Dr. Douglass who wrote: "Pneumococcal bacteremia is an infection of the blood with the bacterium, pneumococcus. It is not a pneumonia and so not subject to vaccine prevention. It is a secondary infection which may, or may not, have come from the lungs."

In that same e-Alert I also told you how regular cleaning of the teeth and gums by a dentist, coupled with good oral hygiene at home, is associated with a reduced risk of pneumonia. Bacteria that develop along the gum line often accumulate in the throat, so when your immune system is not performing at an optimal level this can create respiratory problems such as pneumonia.

Dr. Douglass added this note: "H2O2 solution as a mouth wash twice daily is probably the best and cheap too."

According to several sources I found, a mouth wash of H2O2 (hydrogen peroxide) solution is easy to make. Mix one ounce of 35 percent food-grade hydrogen peroxide with 11 ounces of water. For flavoring, a few drops of liquid chlorophyll can be added. But while you're mixing, care should be taken to avoid undiluted hydrogen peroxide coming into contact with the skin.

My thanks to Dr. Douglass for his dental hygiene recommendation and for further emphasizing the apparent uselessness of the pneumonia vaccine.

To Your Good Health,

Jenny Thompson
Health Sciences Institute

Sources:

- "2 Paths of Bayer Drug in 80's: Riskier Type Went Overseas" Walt Bogdanich and Eric Koli, The New York Times, 5/22/03, nytimes.com

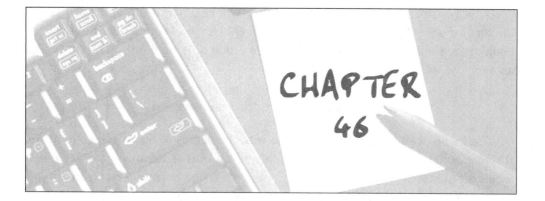

Jumpin' Pax Flash: Paxil prescribed for hot flashes despite laundry list of side effects

First ran 6/9/2003

I was torn. I didn't know whether to laugh or scream. (I guess I did both because a couple of people stopped by my office to see if I was okay.)

That was my reaction last week when I read this "good news" for menopausal women who suffer from hot flashes: A new study concludes that the selective serotonin reuptake inhibitor called paroxetine (better known as Paxil) can reduce the frequency and severity of hot flashes.

This is WONDERFUL news…if you happen to be on the board of directors of GlaxoSmithKline, the makers of Paxil.

But if you're among the many women who will hear about this and ask their doctors for a Paxil prescription, you might eventually find yourself wishing you could trade the Paxil for the hot flashes. The problem is, by then you might not be able to.

3 out of 4 doctors recommend...

There's no need to spend a lot of time with the details of this study, so here are the bare bones: Researchers randomly selected a group of 165 menopausal women who experienced hot flashes and who were not taking a hormone replacement therapy. Roughly one-third of the group received 25 mg of Paxil daily, one-third received 12.5 mg daily, and one-third received a placebo. The frequency and severity of hot flashes were approximately reduced (on average) 65 percent in the first group, 62 percent in the second group, and 38 percent in the placebo group.

The researchers concluded that Paxil may be "an effective and acceptable" therapy for treating hot flashes.

Going just by the numbers of this study, it appears that Paxil does relieve hot flashes. So I'll let them have "effective." But the word I have trouble with is "acceptable." Because given the wide variety of problems that Paxil users have reported over the past decade, it would be stretching the point to call this drug acceptable. And the researchers are certainly well aware of the whole Paxil package because three of the four members of the research team are employees of GlaxoSmithKline.

Nice. I think it was right there I might have screamed.

A good trade off?

Because this study was conducted at Johns Hopkins Medical School, and because it was published in the Journal of the American Medical Association (JAMA), there's no doubt that doctors all over the country will be intoning these prestigious names when assuring their menopausal patients that Paxil is an "effective and acceptable" treatment for their hot flashes.

Acceptable? Here are some of Paxil's side effects described as "frequent": hypertension, impaired concentration, nausea, vomiting, emotional instability, vertigo, inflammation of the mucus membrane, rapid heart beat, weight gain, and temporary suspension of consciousness. And here's my favorite frequent side effect: depression. That's right—the very thing that Paxil is designed to relieve.

What's worse is that some patients report even worse side effects when they try to discontinue their Paxil use. For many years GlaxoSmithKline assured consumers that Paxil was non-habit forming and easy to discontinue. Meanwhile, case after case reported that patients coming off the drug experienced nightmares, dizziness, burning and itching of the skin, agitation, sweating and nausea. And for many of those patients, the only way to treat the side effects was to begin taking Paxil again! And then, just to make it official, last year the FDA issued a warning that withdrawal symptoms from Paxil may be severe.

All of these things are well known about Paxil. So who (other than GlaxoSmithKline employees) could possibly characterize Paxil as an acceptable trade off for hot flashes?

A little spin on the side

ABC television coverage about the JAMA study reported that the researchers "believe" that Paxil is "more promising" than alternative therapies such as vitamin E and black cohosh. Their study had nothing whatsoever to do with any alternative therapies, but ABC kindly helped them create the impression that Paxil trumps natural methods of coping with hot flashes. Of course, ABC didn't mention the GSK connection to the study. They wouldn't want to offend a drug manufacturer that buys plenty of TV advertising for its other products, including Gaviscon, Contac, Tums, Tagament, Flonase, Zantac, Nicorette, and Aquafresh toothpaste.

In an e-Alert I sent you last month ("Spin This" 5/29/03), I told you about a number of alternative therapies that have relieved menopause symptoms for HSI members. Contrary to what the Johns Hopkins researchers would have ABC believe, many women find black cohosh to be very effective in controlling hot flashes. And if black cohosh doesn't work, there are other safe and natural methods to try, including red clover, wild yam progesterone cream, indium sulfate, and vitamin E. (One member wrote to tell us that daily doses of 2000 mg of vitamin C and 400 IU of vitamin E reduced her frequency of hot flashes from 10 each day, to only one. Side effects: none.)

...and another thing

You may have heard how the Atkins diet succeeded in two "controlled" trials, as reported last month in the New England Journal of Medicine (NEJM). An HSI member named Adam heard, and sent these comments:

"It is a shame that the results of the study shows no weight change after a year. There are too many drop outs for the statistics to be non biased. Would like to see your comments."

While the results of these studies had their drawbacks, the details are not as negative as Adam seems to think.

Both studies (from the University of Pennsylvania) compared the Atkins high-protein diet to a high-carbohydrate/low-fat diet in obese subjects. In both trials (one lasted 6 months, and the other a year) the Atkins groups lost more weight than the high-carb groups. In the year-long study, participants of both groups gained back some of their initial weight loss. The authors of the study called the differences between the final net weight losses of the two groups "statistically insignificant." And that's true. But in the end, the Atkins group lost more than the high-carb group.

This may not sound like a resounding success, but it's a success just the same. Because until just recently very few mainstream nutrition or dietary experts would have ever imagined that in a one-year controlled trial a high-protein diet could succeed over a low-fat diet. "Low fat equals good health" has been the mainstream mantra for more than 20 years, but with these studies and others, that mantra is being challenged like never before.

And while it's true that there were dropouts in each of the groups in both studies (as there are in virtually all long-term dietary trials—especially with obese subjects), the dropouts were not so many that the test results were invalidated.

Beyond the fact that the Atkins diet clearly bested the high-carb diet, these equally important results stand out as well: In the one-year trial, the Atkins group had a significantly greater increase in HDL cholesterol, and their triglyceride levels decreased more than in the high-carb group. Similar results occurred in the 6-month trial, with the Atkins group showing greater triglyceride reduction and increased insulin sensitivity compared to the other group.

I think we're so used to seeing wild claims on TV ads ("I lost 50 pound in two days!") that the results of a controlled, year-long trial like this may not seem impressive. In fact, these are very important mainstream successes for a diet that was almost universally dismissed by the nutritional establishment for 30 years.

Somewhere Dr. Atkins is smiling.

To Your Good Health,

Jenny Thompson
Health Sciences Institute

Sources:

- "Paroxetine Controlled Release in the Treatment of Menopausal Hot Flashes" Journal of the American Medical Association, 2003;289;2827-2834, jama.ama-assn.org

- "Frequent Paxil (Paroxetine) Side Effects" Prozac Truth, prozactruth.com

- "Withdrawal From Paroxetine Can Be Severe, Warns FDA" Alison Tonks, British Medical Journal, 2002;324:260, 2/2/02, bmj.com

- "Halting Hot Flashes—Researchers Say Antidepressants May Help Menopausal Women" ABC News, John McKenzie, 6/3/03, abcnews.com

- "A Randomized Trial of a Low-Carbohydrate Diet for Obesity" New England Journal of Medicine, 348:2082-2090, No. 21, 5/22/03, content.nejm.org

- "Atkins Diet Bolstered by Two New Studies" Janet McConnaughey, Associated Press, 5/21/02

- "Atkins' Gains Upper Hand in 'Controlled' Trial" NaturalIngredients.com, 5/22/03, naturalingredients.com

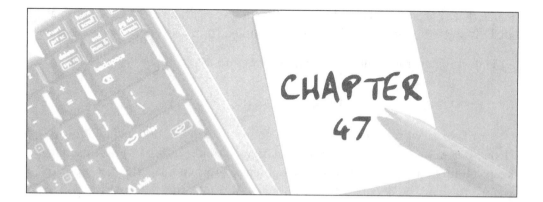

Happy meal: Government OK's releasing previously infected beef into the food supply

First ran 7/29/2003

Would you like to participate in an experiment? There's just one catch: you, your family, and your friends and neighbors are going to be the guinea pigs. Enjoy!

If that sounds like a joke, you won't be laughing when you hear the new information about irradiated meat that appears in the August 2003 issue of Consumer Reports (CR) magazine.

Longtime e-Alert readers know that I have occasionally taken Consumer Reports research to task whenever I felt it veered outside its zone of competence in healthcare matters. But I'll be the first to acknowledge when CR research stays inside that zone and gets it right—which is the case with a recent CR microbial analysis and taste test of irradiated meat sampled from grocery stores in 11 states.

Unfortunately the results don't smell very good.

Suddenly, I'm not hungry

Last February I sent you two e-Alerts about the dangers of irradiated meat: "Don't Beam Me Up" (2/4/03), and "Radiation Nation" (2/10/03). I promised to keep you up to date on the latest developments, so when I saw this CR report I wanted to share the details with you, along with some other information you won't find in the report.

To briefly recap: Irradiation is a process by which a food product is exposed to extremely high doses of radiation that breaks down chemical bonds, killing bacteria, parasites and funguses that may cause disease. But like any technology that monkeys around with nature, you usually end up doing as much damage as good.

Consumer Reports asked specially trained shoppers to purchase grocery store samples of irradiated beef and chicken in 60 U.S. cities. More than 500 samples were cold-packed and shipped to labs for examination. To no one's surprise, the bacteria levels were found to be "significantly" lower in the irradiated meat samples compared to non-irradiated meat. And if that were all that mattered, the test would be a triumph for irradiation.

Two key points from the CR microbial analysis stand out:

1) After meat has been irradiated it can still become contaminated if not handled properly. And according to the Centers for Disease Control, 20 percent of food-borne illnesses are caused by mishandling after meat reaches the store.

2) After meat is purchased, if it's properly stored and cooked, irradiation offers no benefit because proper cooking kills more bacteria than irradiation.

But there's one more point on the safety issue that completely floored me. Here's how the CR report puts it: "The government considers irradiation so effective that it allows tainted ground beef that otherwise would be unlawful to sell, such as meat containing E. coli O157:H7, to be irradiated and sold to consumers."

Staggering, isn't it? Knowing that, and given the choice between irradiated meat and normally processed meat, which would you choose?

Tainted never tasted so good

Selling the idea of irradiated food to consumers has been an uphill battle. The word "irradiated" is a little too close to "radiation" for comfort. So last year congress included a clause in the 2002 Farm Act that broadened the definition of pasteurization. This change was specifically designed so that meat processors and retailers could use the term "cold pasteurized" rather than "irradiation."

But another even more convenient way to ease consumers' fears is to simply mislead them.

The Consumer Reports research discovered two promotional statements for irradiated meat to be untrue. A flyer from one supermarket chain stated that irradiation "eliminates any bacteria that might exist in food." The CR report established that this is untrue, but this was a known fact long before the current issue of CR hit the stands. But it also gives the impression that the meat can't be contaminated, which could easily lead to lax handling and cooking by consumers.

The second statement comes from a pamphlet put out by SureBeam, one of the leading food irradiators. The claim: "You can't taste the difference."

Well...not quite, says CR. According to CR's taste test in which tasters were not aware if they were eating normal or irradiated meat, the irradiated beef and chicken samples were picked out by the tasters in well over half the matchups. The irradiated meat had what was described as a "slight but distinct off taste and smell," and was compared to the aroma of singed hair.

Yum! Would you like a side of E. coli with that?

You are what you irradiate

In his "Daily Dose" e-letter, William Campbell Douglass, M.D., noted another problem with irradiation. In "Zap! Your food is safe" (8/16/02), Dr. Douglass wrote,

"If irradiated food is subsequently mishandled...and becomes contaminated with a disease-causing organism, the food will lack the competing beneficial organisms that could otherwise inhibit its growth. This is comparable to the situation in your intestine. There are trillions of bacteria in your gut, but they are friendly agents when in that environment. If you were to irradiate your gut, you would kill these organisms and there would be a foreign invasion that would probably kill you."

And as if all of that weren't enough, last year a German study showed that a "unique byproduct" created when fat is irradiated may have promoted tumor development in laboratory animals. Further studies were called for and are apparently underway. In response, the European Union has suspended the irradiation of beef and other foods (except for certain spices and herbs) until research can demonstrate that irradiation is safe.

What a concept! Start with thorough testing. THEN, if safety is completely assured, proceed with the technology. Gee, why didn't WE think of that?

In a New York Times article about irradiation last year, Carol Tucker Foreman (the director of the Food Policy Institute at the Consumer Federation of America) stressed the uncertain health risks of irradiation, saying, "There is nowhere in the world where a large population has eaten large amounts of irradiated food over a long period of time."

In other words, every time someone picks up a package of irradiated ground beef at their neighborhood grocery, and every time they order chicken or steak from a restaurant that buys irradiated meat, they're participating in an experiment they didn't even know they signed up for.

At least this way, SureBeam and other irradiation companies don't have to waste a lot of money buying laboratory guinea pigs.

...and another thing

My timing was perfect.

In last Thursday's e-Alert, "Screen Pattern" (7/24/03), I told you why men and their doctors should NOT be quick to proceed with a prostate cancer biopsy based on a single prostate-specific antigen (PSA) screening. A new study shows that fluctuation in PSA levels are responsible for many unnecessary biopsies—painful procedures with unpleasant side effects.

That very same day, the New England Journal of Medicine (NEJM) released a study concluding that PSA screening misses too many cancers. The researchers' recommendation: Lower the acceptable PSA level from 4.0 to 2.6. In other words: Let the biopsies roll!

This is the worst kind of mainstream thinking. With blinders firmly in place, the only reasonable solution these researchers could come up with—in response to a clearly insufficient test—was to sharply INCREASE the number of biopsies. With misguided logic like this, next they'll be saying men should forget about the test altogether and just have a yearly biopsy!

Oh come on! It only hurts for a month!

Fortunately, cooler heads prevailed. In an accompanying NEJM editorial, the authors expressed reservations about the simplistic advice, stating that the recommendation should not yet be accepted as "routine clinical practice." This point was also stressed by doctors on various news programs.

You have to wonder though; in spite of the call to show restraint, will this study just encourage those doctors who already have a "slash and burn" mentality about prostate biopsies? It very well could.

Late Thursday night on my local news, the anchor tucked the PSA study into a 20-second feature toward the end of the broadcast. After calling PSA screening "the gold standard" of prostate cancer testing, he simplified the matter by saying that doctors now recommend that more men receive prostate cancer biopsies.

He was doing his job; cutting the story down to its essential details. But I wonder if he has any idea what damage that sort of sloppy reporting can do when men take the bad advice at face value.

To Your Good Health,

Jenny Thompson
Health Sciences Institute

Sources:

- "Irradiated Meat: Safer But A Little Off—Consumer Group Says Irradiated Meat Not as Safe or Tasty as Claimed" Daniel DeNoon, WebMD Medical News, 7/9/03, content.health.msn.com

- "The Truth About Irradiated Meat" Consumer Reports, August 2003, consumerreports.org

- "How We Tested Beef and Chicken" Consumer Reports, August 2003, consumerreports.org

- "Zap! Your Food is Safe" William Campbell Douglass, M.D., The Daily Dose, 8/16/02, realhealthnews.com

- "Effect of Verification Bias on Screening for Prostate Cancer by Measurement of Prostate-Specific Antigen" New England Journal of Medicine, 349:335-342, No. 4, 7/24/03, content.nejm.org

- "Verification Bias and the Prostate-Specific Antigen Test—Is There a Case for a Lower Threshold for Biopsy?" Fritz H. Schroder, M.D., Ph.D., and Ries Kranse, Ph.D., New England Journal of Medicine, 349:393-395, No. 4, 7/24/03, content.nejm.org

- Prostate Test May Miss Many Tumors" Reuters, 7/23/03, msnbc.com

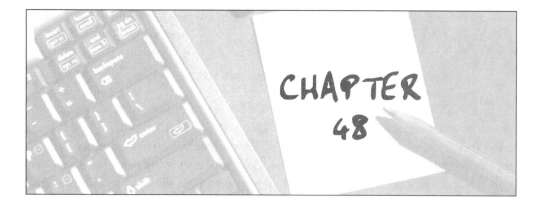

How much is that doctor in the window? Sales practices of the drug companies

First ran 8/11/2003

In "what may be one of the biggest medical deceptions in history," NBC Dateline recently examined the story of a doctor who blew the whistle on the sales practices of a large drug company. But this doctor wasn't on the receiving end of a sales pitch, he was doing the pitching; helping salespeople promote a particular drug for off-label uses…until his conscience got the better of him.

This is a case I first told you about last year in "The Whistle Blower" (6/6/03). At that time, the revelations were astonishing—nothing less than a drug company caught holding a smoking gun. In this new report, additional details emerge that reveal even uglier evidence of what happens when corporate greed is placed way ahead of patient safety.

Hear that lonesome whistle blow

In 1997, Dr. David P. Franklin contacted a lawyer to file suit against his employer, the pharmaceutical company, Warner-Lambert (W-L). Dr. Franklin told the New York Times last year, "I was terrified." Executives at Warner-Lambert had threatened to make him a scapegoat if he went public with his concerns about certain company practices that Dr. Franklin describes as "an illegal marketing scheme that put patients at risk."

Throughout most of the '90s Warner-Lambert (acquired by Pfizer in 2000) manufactured a prescription drug called Neurontin, approved by the FDA for the very specific use of helping to control epileptic seizures for patients already taking another epilepsy drug. But the marketing geniuses at W-L had much bigger plans for Neurontin. So they enlisted people like Dr. Franklin to help drug salespeople convince doctors that Neurontin was useful for a wide range of health problems. (It's not illegal for a doctor to prescribe a drug for conditions it hasn't been approved for, but it is illegal for drug companies to promote off-label use where there's no evidence that the drug is safe or effective for that alternate use.)

In a voice-mail message that's now entered as evidence in Dr. Franklin's lawsuit, a W-L executive told sales reps that in order to make Neurontin profitable they would have to promote it for a variety of off-label uses, such as pain relief, bipolar disorder, and other psychiatric uses, including ADHD for children.

But independent researchers say that Neurontin simply doesn't work for some of those conditions. For instance, when NBC asked a doctor who specializes in bipolar treatment if treating a bipolar patient with Neurontin meant that they were "essentially untreated," the doctor replied, "I think that's a fair assumption." Furthermore, if used inappropriately, Neurontin can cause serious adverse reactions. (The Dateline report tells of one bipolar patient whose doctor simply kept upping the dosage when the patient didn't respond. After becoming uncharacteristically hostile and eventually attempting suicide, she was taken off the Neurontin.)

Little details like that, however, didn't slow down the gung-ho W-L sales team.

After Dr. Franklin became convinced that what he was being asked to do was illegal, he began taping phone conversations and messages, one of which caught this stunning quote from a W-L senior executive: "I don't want to hear that safety crap either...it's a great drug."

This tunnel-vision sales policy seems to have paid off. Since its introduction 10 years ago, Neurontin has become a bonanza, bringing in more than $2 billion each year. Pfizer estimates that off-label use makes up over 75 percent of Neurontin sales.

Is there an ethic in the house?

Part of Neurontin's success may be attributed to the fact that many of the W-L sales reps went much further than simply encouraging doctors to prescribe the drug for off-label use. They crossed the line, and they crossed it arm in arm with quite a few doctors who did something completely unprofessional and inexcusable.

In a so-called "shadowing program," W-L paid 75 to 100 doctors for allowing sales reps to sit in during patient exams. This invasion of privacy, condoned by doctors who were trusted by their patients, is nothing less than deplorable.

At the conclusion of the exams the sales reps gave "recommendations" on what medicines to prescribe. The doctors were paid $350 or more for each day the sales people were allowed to spend in the exam rooms. Hundreds of patients were affected by this program, but whether or not any of them knew that the person sitting in for their exam was a pharmaceutical salesperson is unclear.

More than one out of three doctors

Can it get any worse? Sure it can.

Court documents accuse Warner-Lambert of hiring a marketing firm to write medical journal articles that would place Neurontin in a positive light. W-L is said to have paid $12,000 for each article, as well as an additional $1,000 to various doctors who agreed to allow their names to be listed as "authors." Salespeople were then able to distribute the not-quite-kosher articles to doctors to help persuade them that Neurontin was safe and effective for off-label uses.

Dr. Franklin's case also shows that doctors who prescribed high volumes of Neurontin were rewarded with additional payments for "consulting" or "speaking" fees.

As I've noted in previous e-Alerts, these sorts of sales tactics have become business as usual for the giant drug companies that spend billions of dollars encouraging physicians to prescribe certain products. In fact, 37 percent of the doctors who participated in a 2002 Maryland survey said they had accepted compensation from drug companies in return for prescribing their drugs.

And guess who helped pay for many of those prescriptions? Dr. Franklin's lawsuit has led to a federal investigation claiming that Medicaid paid tens of millions of dollars for Neurontin prescriptions written for untested uses. Those were our tax dollars at work for Warner-Lambert!

Profiting ugly

Today, Dr. Franklin—a former research fellow at Harvard Medical School—is the director of market research at Boston Scientific, a company that develops medical devices. Reflecting on his time at Warner-Lambert, he says the thing that was most troubling was the pressure they put on him to encourage doctors to prescribe Neurontin in much higher doses than it was approved for. He told the New York Times, "I recognized that my actions may be putting people in harm's way."

And Pfizer, through a spokesperson, offers this defense of the ongoing legal mess: "The actions that allegedly occurred took place well before Pfizer completed its merger with Warner-Lambert. It is firm and established Pfizer policy not to allow our sales representatives to make inappropriate claims or encourage off-label use of any of our medicines."

So are we really supposed to believe that Warner-Lambert's sales policy for Neurontin was just an isolated case in an industry that's otherwise honest and has our best interests in mind? The answer to that depends on who you choose to believe: an international drug company spokesperson, or a whistle blower who saw from the inside just how ugly the business of selling prescription drugs can be.

...and another thing

It's sticky and steamy in London.

Last week, I received an e-mail from a colleague named Rachael in HSI's London office. Rachael wrote to tell me about, "a ludicrous report from a leading UK newspaper (The Times), which warns that the Atkins diet is unsafe to follow in hot weather (there's currently a heat wave in the UK...makes a change!!)"

Rachael kindly included the Times article, which quoted Dr. Sarah Schenker, a dietician and spokesman for the British Nutrition Foundation. Dr. Schenker told the Times, "The body has to work harder to metabolise protein than other food types. This means that on a really hot day, people on the protein-based diet who are facing, say, the Underground could have problems. My advice would be avoid the Atkins diet in hot weather."

Dr. Schenker seems to be unaware that the Atkins diet is not simply one plate of T-bones and pork chops after another. In fact, many fruits and vegetables are low in carbohydrates and can be eaten while following the Atkins plan.

Meanwhile, we've seen how a heavy intake of carbohydrates can contribute to obesity. And it's quite obvious that obese people have a very hard time of it during extremely hot weather. If Dr. Schenker has any warm weather menu suggestions for the obese or anyone else, she didn't share them with the Times. I guess she just showed up to bash Atkins, and then took off to find the nearest air conditioner and a heaping plate of pasta.

If you're wondering how popular the Atkins diet is in the UK, here's a good indicator: The only book that "Dr. Atkins' New Diet Revolution" is currently NOT outselling is the new Harry Potter.

I wonder if J.K. Rowling has considered writing a Harry Potter diet book? She might end up with an even bigger following than Dr. Atkins.

To Your Good Health,

Jenny Thompson
Health Sciences Institute

Sources:

- "Drug Giant Accused of False Claims" NBC Dateline, 7/11/03, msnbc.com
- "Suit Says Company Promoted Drug in Exam Rooms" The New York Times, 5/15/02, nytimes.com
- "Health Warning to Atkins Dieters as the Heat Goes on" Sam Coates and Patrick Barkham, The Times of London, 8/7/03, timesonline.co.uk

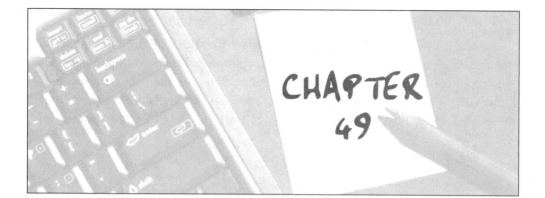

Does this smell bad? The nasal flu spray vaccine

First ran 12/10/2003

You've probably heard the news by now: Doctors are running low on flu vaccines and are expected to run out completely before the flu season winds down. In one of the TV reports I saw, the commentator asked, "How could this happen?" And I had to laugh.

How could it happen?

Hmmm…let's put on our thinking caps and try real hard to figure it out. Could it possibly be because nearly every TV news broadcast for the past month has been saying that this will be the worst flu season in years and everyone needs to drop what they're doing—RIGHT NOW!—and go get a flu shot?

Making this news all the more dire is the fact that the final drop of flu vaccine has already been shipped out, so once the vaccine supply is used up, no more vaccine can be produced until next year. But before you barricade yourself in your home,vowing to stay safe inside until the flu season has passed, rest assured that there JUST HAPPENS to be an alternative to the dwindling vaccine supplies.

Come and get it!

Remember FluMist? It's the nasal-spray flu vaccine I first told you about in the e-Alert "Nose Candy" (7/8/03). Unlike the conventional flu shot, which contains inactivated flu strains, FluMist contains three living flu strains. The Centers for Disease Control (CDC) calls FluMist "live attenuated influenza vaccine" or LAIV. In other words, the three strains are diluted. They're alive as you or me, but watered down.

Now—a show of hands—how many would feel comfortable inhaling not one, not two, but THREE LIVING flu strains? Not too many, is my guess. Which is probably one of the main reasons why ABC News has described sales of FluMist as "disappointing." Disappointing so far, anyway.

According to the Washington Post, the CDC gave FluMist a nice little boost last week when a statement was released "reminding" the public that FluMist is an appropriate alternative to the flu shot for those who are both healthy and between the ages of 5 and 49. Then on Monday, CDC director Dr. Julie Gerberding made appearances on several national news broadcasts (including ABC and CNN) and mentioned that a large supply of FluMist is still available.

Now is it just me and my cynical streak, or does it seem somehow to be a very, let's say "interesting," coincidence that the country has been plunged into this supposedly dire emergency of vaccine shortage in the same year that a major new vaccine product is launched? No one I know has said they haven't been able to get a flu shot. And I haven't read about any doctors turning away patients who have requested a shot. But if the CDC says the supply is low, then I suppose the supply is low. And if the CDC says that the supply of FluMist is high, then I'm sure the supply is high.

What Dr. Gerberding didn't mention is that FluMist costs more than twice the amount of the flu shot. And because of this much steeper cost, many insurance companies won't offer coverage for FluMist. But that's only part of the FluMist problem.

Pig in a poke

As I stated in the July e-Alert, there's a long list of potential problems with FluMist, but one of the key problems is the fact that those who decide to sniff living viruses into their heads instantly become infected by the flu. The immune system then responds by creating more antibodies that, in theory, will fight off any full-strength flu strains that might come along. But in the meantime, there's a possibility that those who are recently FluMisted could be (I'll bet you already guessed it) contagious!

Nice. Just what we need in the middle of a supposed flu epidemic: more contagious people running around.

Of course, the makers of FluMist (MedImmune, a subsidiary of the drug giant Wyeth) play down the possibility of their product spreading the flu, stating that only a very small percentage of FluMist users will actually transmit a virus. Nevertheless, according to a report in Knight-Ridder Newspapers, the CDC cautions those who get a FluMist vaccine to stay away from people with vulnerable immune systems, such as the elderly or those struggling with diseases, for one week. But is one week long enough? Some hospitals are telling their personnel to allow three full weeks between their FluMist vaccine and contact with hospital patients.

Why the discrepancy? My guess is that this is such a new vaccine that no one really knows the parameters yet. Nevertheless, the CDC seems to be going out of their way to help MedImmune move their struggling product.

Add to that; the CDC web site states: "The optimal time to receive influenza vaccine is usually in October or November." So if they're using the same calendar I'm using, we're already 10 days past the optimal usage period.

And add to that; the people who supposedly need a flu vaccine the most—the elderly, and those with immune system diseases—shouldn't be taking FluMist at all. The FDA hasn't approved it for them. So the CDC is pressing those who are least vulnerable to the flu to run out and get a snootful of this expensive and relatively untested product, even though it's almost two weeks past the optimal timing for the vaccine to even work!

Does any of this smell bad to you?

Bouncing back

Without question, many are going to come down with the flu or some other unpleasant virus this season. Tomorrow I'll leave the cares and woes of vaccines behind to take a look at some of the natural treatments that can help you kick a viral illness, while giving your immune system every advantage to do its best work.

And they even work in December!

...and another thing

Normally I'm not a bit shy about putting in my 2 cents on a topic. In fact, I've kept a huge penny collection handy ever since I spoke my first words. But today I'm going to up the ante and put in my 10 cents...

In 1937, the National Foundation for Infantile Paralysis was established by President Franklin Delano Roosevelt to raise funds for polio research. Eddie Cantor, a popular comedian of the time, asked audiences to donate dimes to the foundation. This drive was referred to as the "March of Dimes," which the foundation later adopted as its name. In 1946, FDR's profile was added to the dime to memorialize a president of great compassion who was credited for guiding the U.S. out of an economic depression and through a World War. No small potatoes.

But then came the miniseries.

I'm sure you heard about all the ruckus raised when CBS tried to air a miniseries last month that portrayed President Ronald Reagan in an unflattering light. In a miffed response, Representative Mark Souder of Indiana introduced the "Ronald Reagan Dime Act" which proposes to replace FDR's dime profile with Reagan's. Rep. Souder has signed up 89 co-sponsors for the bill.

Personally I think it's a wonderful idea to find ways to honor Ronald Reagan. But there are ways to honor him without deliberately taking an honor away from another great president. And it certainly appears that Rep. Souder and the co-sponsors of the bill seem to believe that President Reagan is somehow more fully honored if a Democratic icon is stripped of his honor.

Speaking out on this clearly partisan act, one critic of the Reagan dime told the Associated Press last week, "It would be wrong to remove him (FDR) and replace him with another. It is my hope that the proposed legislation will be withdrawn." And before you jump to the conclusion that that quote might have come from a certain former first lady who is now a senator, it actually comes from another former first lady, Nancy Reagan, who added that she felt certain her husband would not support the Reagan Dime Act.

I'm behind the Reagans 100 percent on this one.

And that's my 10 cents.

To Your Good Health,

Jenny Thompson
Health Sciences Institute

Sources:

- "Questions and Answers About Live Attenuated Influenza Vaccine (Trade Name FluMist)" Centers for Disease Control, cdc.gov

- "Be Cautious, FluMist Users" Richard Harkness, Knight Ridder Newspapers, 12/4/03, fortwayne.com

- "MedImmune Poised as Flu Spreads" The Washington Post, 12/8/03, washingtonpost.com

- "CDC Director: 'Doing Everything We Can' to Distribute Flu Vaccine" CNN, 12/8/03, cnn.com

- "House Tossup In Dime Design" Jim Geraghty, States News Service, 12/8/03, washingtonpost.com

- "Nancy Reagan Opposes Replacing FDR With Reagan On Dimes" Associated Press, 12/5/03, freerepublic.com

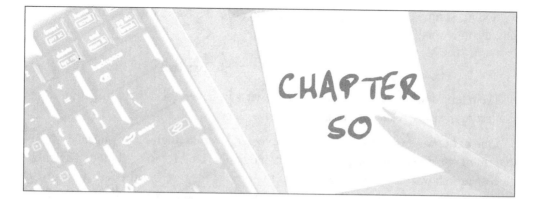

Lucky 7:
The importance of blood
sugar control for diabetics

First ran 12/8/2004

Last month, smack in the middle of Diabetes Awareness Month, a group of health advocates joined 50 U.S. mayors to launch a campaign called "Aim. Believe. Achieve: The Diabetes A1C Initiative."

Here at HSI, we consider every month to be Diabetes Awareness Month. After all, type 2 diabetes is a disease that affects more than 11 million U.S. citizens, but it's estimated that less than half of those 11 million have adequate control of their blood sugar levels. So awareness obviously needs to be a 12-month project.

And that's the crux of the A1C Initiative: to make type 2 diabetics and their doctors aware of a simple test that can help keep close tabs on blood sugar.

Sounds simple enough. Except that according to ABC News the A1C Initiative has raised controversy among many doctors.

The seven percent solution

I've referred to the A1C test in several e-Alerts because researchers sometimes use the test to measure results in trials that involve diabetes.

One of the ways to assess the severity of hyperglycemia (high blood sugar) is to determine the percentage of glycosylated hemoglobin (HbA1c) in the blood. A fasting glucose test shows the blood sugar level at the time of the test, but the A1C test reveals the average measurement of HbA1c percentage in the blood over the 60 to 90 days prior to the test date, providing a much more reliable profile of blood sugar level.

In a nutshell: An HbA1c level of five percent is considered safe, and seven percent or less is considered normal. A level higher than seven is a red flag, signaling the possibility of type 2 diabetes.

The title of the Diabetes A1C Initiative program is "A1C<7% by 2007," and as the name implies, the goal is to encourage as many type 2 diabetics as possible to focus on reaching the 7 percent A1C target for their blood sugar levels over the next two to three years. Getting tested is easy—it only takes a single drop of blood—but it does require a visit to the doctor. Ideally the A1C test should be conducted three or four times each year; especially for those who are at high risk of diabetes or have problems controlling blood sugar levels.

Skeptics collide

So...Where's the controversy in A1C? Apparently only at ABC.

According to an ABC News report that coincided with the A1C Initiative launch, "many doctors are skeptical" about the A1C Initiative. But only two skeptical doctors are quoted in the article. One of them feels that the A1C test is being promoted by "experts" who are affiliated with drug companies. Of course, he doesn't mention that finding an expert, doctor or researcher in mainstream medicine who hasn't been affiliated with a drug company would be as rare as finding a boxcar filled with hens' teeth.

The other skeptic is a doctor and researcher who feels that controlling blood sugar in diabetics is relatively unimportant compared to more pressing issues for diabetics, such as cigarette smoking, blood pressure and the use of the diabetic medication metformin. Yep—amazing but true—he considers the use of metformin to be more important than controlling blood sugar.

Metformin is the most common mainstream medication prescribed to type 2 diabetics. It comes with a black box warning to indicate that the drug has been associated with a condition called lactic acidosis that can have fatal side effects for patients with kidney disease and congestive heart failure. And yet, in spite of that high profile warning, a 2002 study found that as many as one out of four patients who are prescribed metformin have kidney dysfunction, congestive heart failure, or both.

So if there's any real controversy in the ABC article, it's the contradiction between the two doctors who are skeptical about the A1C Initiative—one claiming that it's promoted by drug company interests, and the other emphasizing the importance of drug use over blood sugar control.

Let's get real

Meanwhile, those two skeptical doctors are overlooking one glaringly obvious element of the A1C Initiative: The campaign does not in any way downplay the importance of other health factors that affect diabetics, it simply emphasizes the need to control blood sugar levels—a factor that should not be underestimated.

In the e-Alert "Sugar Shock" (9/28/04), I told you about research from Johns Hopkins University that analyzed the association between heart disease in diabetic subjects and the severity of hyperglycemia. After reviewing 13 individual studies, the Hopkins team concluded that hyperglycemia may be directly associated with an increased risk of heart disease in people with diabetes. The researchers estimated that every time HbA1c increases by one percentage point, the risk of heart disease or stroke raises by nearly 20 percent. Likewise, when HbA1c percentage drops, heart disease risk drops as well.

Without question, all diabetics should quit smoking and pay close attention to other health factors associated with their condition. But to dismiss the importance of blood sugar levels is foolish. Especially when a simple test provides an easy way to monitor this key marker of diabetic health.

...and another thing

Just between you and me

Confidentiality isn't what it used to be

My husband and I recently applied for a new life insurance policy, which required us to take physical exams. And of course, among the paperwork that we filled out there was a confidentiality statement promising that the results of our exams would be strictly private.

When the exam results came back, we weren't surprised when my husband's cholesterol was on the high side. It's been high for awhile now, we've known about it, and he's taking steps to address it (although you can be sure that he's NOT taking a statin drug).

What DID surprise me was something that arrived in the mail just a couple of days later. It was a flier, addressed to my husband, with tips on how to lower cholesterol. The flier was sponsored by a drug company. And it's the first one he's ever received.

Think I hit the ceiling? Uh...YEAH! We're still repairing ceiling tiles.

Our new insurance company agreed not to share our medical exam results with our doctor, the government, our insurance broker, etc. But apparently that confidentiality doesn't extend to drug companies that like to offer friendly "tips" on how to lower cholesterol.

In short, their definition of confidential and mine are somewhat different.

Mine means you keep something in confidence. Theirs means we're confident we can do something valuable with this information.

To Your Good Health,

Jenny Thompson

Health Sciences Institute

Sources:

- "Mayors Campaign Challenges Americans to Achieve Diabetes Control" Press Release, Aim. Believe. Achieve: The Diabetes A1C Initiative" 11/18/04, biz.yahoo.com
- "New Diabetes Campaign Raises Controversy" Ali Mohamadi, ABC News, 11/18/04, abcnews.go.com

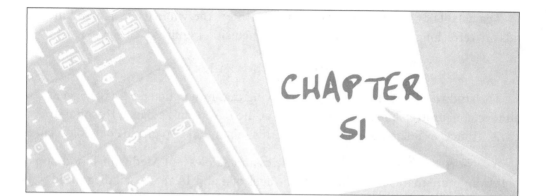

Attention paid: The connection between ADHD and diet

First ran 1/12/2005

You've probably noticed that attention-deficit/hyperactivity disorder (ADHD) has been "re-branded" in the mainstream medical marketplace. Yep—it's not just for kids anymore. If we're to believe the ads, it seems that adults also have problems focusing on details and setting priorities.

With so much media attention devoted to the popular ADHD drugs targeted at this expanding customer base, it's rare to come across an ADHD study that doesn't involve any drugs at all. And even more rare is a study that dares imply that a nutritional deficiency might actually play a role in attention deficit.

Against all odds, however, I found such a study. And while its design and methods are refreshingly drug-free, the dietary conclusion requires a closer look.

Bring on the kids

The study itself is simple enough. Knowing that iron deficiency may trigger abnormal neurotransmission, researchers at the European Pediatric Hospital in Paris, France, evaluated the deficiency of this mineral in two groups of adolescents.

As reported in the Archives of Pediatrics and Adolescent Medicine, blood samples from more than 50 kids between the ages of 4 and 14 years—all diagnosed with ADHD—were examined to determine ferritin levels. (Ferritin is a protein that stores iron.) The researchers also examined blood samples from a control group of nearly 30 kids with no symptoms of ADHD.

The French team reported three striking results:

- The ADHD group had a lower average ferritin level compared to the control group
- Almost 85 percent of the ADHD kids had abnormal ferritin levels, compared to less than 20 percent of the control subjects
- The most severe ADHD symptoms were observed in kids with low ferritin levels

In their conclusion, the researchers write that low iron stores may contribute to ADHD, and children with ADHD might benefit from iron supplementation.

The plus and the minus

I knew that HSI Panelist Allan Spreen, M.D., would find this study interesting. In the e-Alert "How to Dismantle an '89 Ford" (6/3/02), Dr. Spreen wrote at some length about the ways nutrition directly affects kids' behavior, particularly in regard to ADHD.

After looking over the French research, Dr. Spreen told me he thought the results were dependable, and described the study as "very helpful." But he added: "Then again, there's some reading between the lines that I would suggest..."

Dr. Spreen: "Unfortunately, it can be a bit more difficult than just giving iron in such a situation. One of the rubs comes in when you try to evaluate whether the problem is actually iron or could these kids be generally nutritionally deficient? No levels of any other nutrients were taken, so we have no idea at all if the problem is really iron or a plethora of nutrients. (My personal experience leads me to believe that such kids are generally trashed, nutritionally, besides just iron, which is all that ferritin measures.)"

The bigger picture

"Okay, so let's say the problem is iron...alone. Most of the solutions tend to be inorganic iron in supplement form (or, heaven forbid, by injection). First, it tends to be poorly absorbed, and second, such agents are well known to generate the formation of free radicals, molecules that damage cell membranes throughout the body. That's why our bodies insulate us from our own iron by placing it within a heme ring (hemoglobin). We need the stuff for oxygen transfer, but we also need to be protected from it. That's why I recommend organic iron, as in calves liver (good luck getting THAT down a kid), or desiccated liver tablets.

"So the problem is STILL iron. Remember that, free radicals or not, it's possible that the iron may not be absorbed well. I've had several patients who took iron (including painful injections) for laboratory-confirmed anemia (low iron levels) and still remained anemic! When I threw in high levels of vitamin B-12 and folic acid (higher than the silly RDA), even if they were not clinically low in these nutrients, their iron levels normalized. That's why I've learned to take a more 'shotgun' approach, even if I think I know what the actual problem is.

"Ah, but it gets better (or, maybe, worse): I don't think correcting iron alone will do it (with or without B-12, folic acid, and maybe even digestive enzymes). If food allergies are not dealt with, if sugar and refined white flour are not massively lowered, if artificial additives are not eliminated (colors, flavors, MSG, preservatives, etc.), the changes from supplements could still fail to work properly.

"I FIRMLY believe ADHD is fixable...without drugs of any kind in the VAST majority of cases."

If you have a child, a grandchild or a friend who may have been diagnosed with ADHD, I strongly recommend Dr. Spreen's nutritional tips for addressing this problem. To read about them in more detail, you can easily use key words to search for "How to Dismantle an '89 Ford" in the HSI e-Alert archives on our web site: hsibaltimore.com.

...and another thing

Can your diet affect your joints?

A friend of mine with arthritis recently asked me if there were any foods she should stay away from that might aggravate her condition. And in fact there are some foods that can add to joint pain.

Many arthritis sufferers are highly sensitive to solanine, an alkaloid known for its toxicity. Solanine is found in plants called nightshade or deadly nightshade plants. Well known edible nightshade plants include tomatoes, potatoes, green and red peppers, eggplants, and cayenne. Removing these solanine-rich foods from your diet may be a good first step toward eliminating dietary triggers of joint pain; a frequently overlooked element in the treatment of arthritis.

Obviously, a salad with tomatoes and green peppers isn't going to be "deadly," but arthritis patients may find some measure of relief with a reduced intake of nightshade foods.

To Your Good Health,

Jenny Thompson
Health Sciences Institute

Sources:

- "Iron Deficiency in Children With Attention-Deficit/Hyperactivity Disorder" Archives of Pediatrics & Adolescent Medicine, Vol. 158, No. 12, December 2004, ncbi.nlm.nih.gov

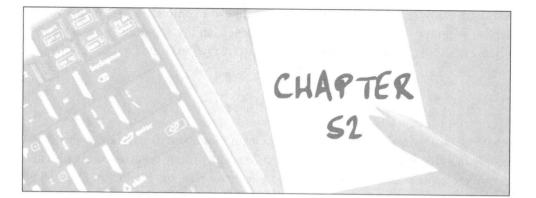

CHAPTER
52

RADAR detector: Is the FDA opposed to better tracking for drug reactions?

First ran 5/16/2005

Out with the new...in with the old.

A large majority of consumers would prefer to take a drug that's been on the market for 10 years or more before trying a newer drug, according to a recent survey conducted by Medco Health Solutions.

You have to wonder; would that same survey have had a completely different outcome five years ago, or even one year ago? In the past few months we've seen some best selling drugs crash and burn amid safety concerns, while major drug companies and the FDA have taken hit after hit in the mainstream media.

And now, at exactly the time the FDA could use a complete image makeover, agency executives have made an astonishing decision that would be no less surprising than if FDA acting commissioner Lester Crawford called a press conference, drew a gun, and actually shot himself in the foot.

Hit and miss

What's the primary job of the FDA? To insure food and drug safety, right? And how is that done? In the case of drugs, FDA executives rely on drug companies and doctors to report adverse reactions. This information is compiled in an FDA database. But gathering the information is only the first step. In some cases it takes several years to analyze the data in order to recognize and respond to a proven adverse reaction.

Under this system drug companies are basically being asked to police themselves. (That would be like asking Tony Soprano to, pretty please, not have anybody "whacked.") But relying on reports of adverse reactions from doctors is also undependable. M.D.s are expected to report adverse reactions on a voluntary basis. But the process is time consuming and in some cases doctors may fear that investigations will draw malpractice suits.

By some estimates more than 90 percent of all adverse reactions go unreported. And yet, according the Chicago Tribune, the FDA receives as many as 400,000 yearly reports of adverse reactions, and the worst of these reactions account for about 100,000 deaths each year.

RADAR network

Five years ago, Northwestern University researchers Charles L. Bennett, M.D., Ph.D., began building a better radar to detect adverse reactions to drugs. In fact, he called his project RADAR: Research for Adverse Drug Events and Reports.

Dr. Bennett's process is fairly simple. Twenty-five doctors from five U.S. cities report their observations of potential adverse reactions, with special interest paid to the most serious reactions that could be fatal. When reports come in they're then sent out to a larger group of researchers who begin to hunt for other reports. The FDA post-marketing database is one of the sources used for additional reporting.

To date, 16 different drugs and medical devices have been linked to adverse reactions that are potentially fatal. RADAR has identified severe adverse reactions in nearly 1,700 patients, and 10 percent of those patients died of complications associated with the reactions.

So has the FDA embraced Dr. Bennett's RADAR? If you guessed "no" to that question, you're on the right track. But even hardened cynics might be surprised at what happened next.

The big dog bites

One of the drugs that RADAR examined was Plavix, a popular clot-prevention drug. According to the Chicago Tribune, Dr. Bennett's researchers reported that in rare cases Plavix may trigger a "catastrophic collapse of the blood system." At Dr. Bennett's urging the FDA added a warning to the drug packaging.

Dr. Bennett followed up the Plavix research with a study that compared how four years of adverse reactions to Plavix were tracked by the FDA, Bristol-Myers Squibb (BMS, the makers of Plavix) and the RADAR team. As reported in the February 2004 issue of the journal Stroke, Dr. Bennett scored RADAR's effectiveness at 92 to 100 percent, while BMS scored between 8 to 58 percent and the FDA scored zero to 23 percent. Dr. Bennett gave the FDA a failing grade.

The FDA's response? Apparently, someone at the agency was not very pleased. The Tribune reports that FDA officials reacted to the Stroke study by terminating Dr. Bennett's access to the agency's database.

The 16 to watch

Earlier this month the Journal of the American Medical Association published the RADAR conclusions of Dr. Bennett and his colleagues. The study included a list of these 16 drugs and medical devices that have produced adverse effects: Zolendronate, Amiodarone, Epoetin, Thalidomide, Gerncitabine, Ticiopidine, Gerntuzumab, Clopidogrel, Nevirapine, Flutamide, Sirolimus-eluting cardiac stent, rHu-MGDF (for thrombocytopenia), Bicalutamide, Enoxaparin, rHu-MGDF (for lymphomas), Paclitaxel-eluting cardiac stent.

If you're currently using any of these drugs or devices, or if you know someone who is, it would be wise to talk to your doctor about the potential risks. But make sure he's not relying on the FDA's data.

...and another thing

Time travel is bad for your health.

That's my theory, anyway. I'm guessing that all future attempts to travel back and forth through time will turn out to have dire side effects. Otherwise folks from the future would be as common as reality TV show contestants.

The adverse side effect problem might also explain why no time travelers showed up at the Massachusetts Institute of Technology Time Traveler Convention last week. But you can't say the MIT conventioneers didn't give it their best effort when it came to publicizing the event.

Imagining that all the kinks of time travel might not be worked out for perhaps thousands of years, they proposed ways to publish convention details in "enduring forms."

In other words, they weren't just trying to get a good turnout—they wanted to make time travelers from the far off future aware of their convention in hopes that so many of them might show up it would become a "Woodstock-like event that defines humanity forever."

I wonder if they planned ahead to provide parking for 500,000 time machines.

So how do you send an invitation to someone many centuries in the future? Not with a web site. Sooner or later the Internet will be an outmoded curiosity. The convention planners' suggestions: "Write the details down on a piece of acid-free paper, and slip them into obscure books in academic libraries! Carve them into a clay tablet!"

If anyone actually tried these methods, they didn't seem to work. But here's a thought: Maybe someone carved a clay tablet, but when the time travelers didn't show up, destroyed the tablet after the convention because it obviously hadn't gotten the message through, but maybe the reason it didn't get through was because the tablet was destroyed, so if the tablet hadn't been destroyed...

I'm getting dizzy just thinking about it. A perfect example of how time travel can create health problems.

To Your Good Health,

Jenny Thompson
Health Sciences Institute

Sources:

- "Americans Prefer 'Safer' Older Drugs" Reuters Health, 5/6/05, reutershealth.com

- "The Research on Adverse Drug Events and Reports (RADAR) Project" Journal of the American Medical Association, Vol. 293, No. 17, 5/4/05, jama.ama-assn.org

- "RADAR Detects Sometimes-Deadly Drug Reactions" Elizabeth Weise, USA Today, 5/3/05, usatoday.com

- "FDA Cut Off Critic's Access to Drug Database" Ronald Kotulak, Chicago Tribune, 2/20/05, chicagotribune.com

- "We Need Your Help For the Time Traveler Convention" Massachusetts Institute of Technology, 5/7/05, web.mit.edu

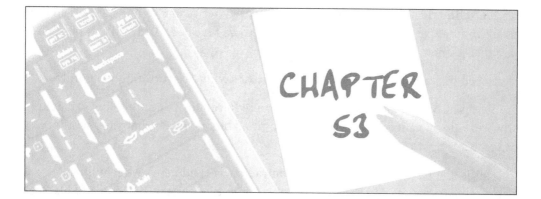

Compression obsession: Doing away with mammograms

First ran 6/7/2005

Women of Detroit, Michigan…I've got good news for you.

Women of Boston, Houston, New York and 12 other cities in the U.S., Canada and Europe, I've got good news for you too.

And for women who don't live in any of these cities, I hope to have some very good news for you as well in about a year and a half when we'll get the results of a trial that will hopefully do away with mammograms forever.

You're going to WHAT?

Women who go to a radiology clinic for their first mammogram are often surprised to find that their breasts must be squeezed between two flat surfaces so the tissue will be sparse enough to allow tumors to be revealed. And you can be certain that it's not a tender squeeze.

To call this "uncomfortable" is a nice way of saying "excruciatingly painful."

But it's also dangerous. The compression required for mammograms can actually break down cancer tissue and rupture small blood vessels that support the cancer, causing it to spread.

This is known as the "compression contradiction," and here's what William Campbell Douglass II, M.D., had to say about it in the January 2002 issue of his Real Health Breakthroughs Newsletter: "I find it maddeningly contradictory that medical students are taught to examine breasts gently to keep any possible cancer from spreading, yet radiologists are allowed to manhandle them for a mammogram."

When Dr. Douglass says "manhandle," that's a nice way of saying "squashed flat."

Three up...three down

Whenever I write about mammograms I always receive messages from women who feel they owe their lives to cancer detected by mammograms. I don't doubt that at all, but I still believe that mammograms will someday be viewed as barbaric and ineffective.

In the e-Alert "Easy as 1...2...3" (8/5/03), I told you about three mammography myths:

1) Mammograms are safe. In fact, they're not. Compression of the breast may prompt cancer to spread. And then there's the radiation: A mammogram delivers about 1,000 times more radiation than a chest x-ray and carries a risk of cardiovascular damage.

2) Mammograms catch cancer at an early stage. In fact, if a tumor is large enough to be detected by a mammogram it's most likely already in an advanced state.

3) Mammograms save lives. In fact, studies have shown that women who have mammograms suffer about the same rate of death due to breast cancer as women who do not have mammograms.

For many more details about these three myths, you can find the e-Alert "Easy as 1...2...3" on our web site at hsibaltimore.com.

Reading the currents

Mammography is not the future of breast cancer detection. And I've got a feeling that even proponents of mammography would agree with that.

In the e-Alert "Firing Back" (8/13/03), I told you about an experimental technique called computed tomography laser mammography (CTLM); a breast imaging system that uses a combination of laser light and thermal heat (but no radiation) to produce a full color, three-dimensional cross-section view of each breast. This method—which is quick and painless—is still being developed and tested.

Today we'll turn our attention to another new technique called the Breast Cancer Detection System (BCDS); a method that's also completely non-invasive and radiation-free. And best of all: no squashing.

Hear that sound? That's the sound of female HSI members shouting in unison: "Halleluiah!"

BCDS technology is based on the discovery that electricity passes through cancerous tissue differently than it passes through normal tissue. A BCDS device consists of several strips containing electronic sensors that are laid over the breast in a spoke-like pattern. Very low electrical currents are transmitted into the breast without causing any pain to the patient. Diagnosis is made with computer analysis.

A South Carolina company called Z-tech is now conducting the final stage of clinical trials with an 18-month test of BCDS at 16 medical centers in the U.S., Canada and Europe. And you can be sure that this is a trial I'll be following very closely.

If you'd like to find out if one of the BCDS test sites is located in your area, just go to the Z-Tech web site at z-techinc.com and select "Clinical Trials." Needless to say, I'd be very interested to hear from anyone who contacts one of these test sites and joins the trial.

...and another thing

An apple a day may not keep the doctor away, but it will deliver plenty of antioxidant-rich polyphenols that help prevent and fight chronic diseases.

Now we find that the type of daily apple you choose may make a big difference.

Researchers at Agriculture and Agri-Food Canada tested eight different species of apple to measure polyphenol activity. The species included Northern Spy, Golden Delicious, Red Delicious, Empire, Cortland, McIntosh, Mutsu and Ida Red. All the apples used in the study were grown on the same farm.

The results:

- Red Delicious, Northern Spy and Ida Red apples had the highest levels of polyphenol activity
- Red Delicious had twice the polyphenol activity than Empire apples, which had the least
- Polyphenols are far more concentrated in the apple peel than the flesh of the apple

According to previous research, a single apple has antioxidant activity that is roughly equal to 1,500 mg of vitamin C. Provided, of course, you choose wisely when you go apple picking.

To Your Good Health,

Jenny Thompson
Health Sciences Institute

Sources:

- "Detecting Breast Cancer" Matt McMillen, The Washington Post, 5/3/05, washingtonpost.com
- "Red Delicious Apples Packed with Disease Fighting Antioxidants" Lindsey Partos, NutraIngredients.com, 5/25/05, nutraingredients.com

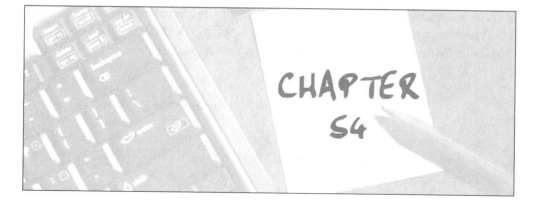

The good doctor: Doctor's license revoked for practicing alternative medicine

First ran 6/30/2005

Imagine finding a doctor who seemed able to heal almost any problem you had—from a back in complete spasm to a sinus infection. Add to that the fact that he would spend 30, 45, even 90 minutes taking care of you—not letting you leave the office until your pain was gone. But wait, it gets even better. Because he spends so much time with each patient, his office encourages you to call before you come so you don't spend too much time waiting and reading old magazines rather than actually accomplishing something.

So here we have a doctor who cares about actually helping patients, is capable of truly healing them, and knows their time is valuable. What would you do if you found such an amazing doctor? If you were the State of Maryland Board of Physicians (MBP), the answer is simple: you would revoke his license to practice medicine.

If he sinks, he's innocent…

So surely, this man whom I so admire, must have done something criminal or at least negligent. Patients must have been complaining, suffering or maybe dying. After all, they don't just randomly pull doctors out of practice.

Apparently, they do.

For years, the MBP has had Binyamin C. Rothstein, D.O., on probation for the crime of practicing alternative and complementary medicine. Without a single patient complaint, his treatment methods were deemed inappropriate by peer review.

During his probationary period, they ordered him to shut down his chelation practice—and he did. They demanded patient records, and they got them. (Dr. Rothstein's assistant told me the records didn't include the original form filled out by the patient because she thought that was privileged. Do we have a jail secure enough for this dangerous Bonnie and Clyde duo?!)

The only specific treatment he continued that the MBP had cited him for was…using IV vitamin cocktails. Oh, the horror! I hope there are no children in the room that might be reading this.

Sliding scales of justice

To give you the complete perspective of how grave these violations were, let me tell you about some of the other doctors who were disciplined by the MBP last month.

One of them had his license revoked because he was convicted of second-degree murder. Another doctor received only a suspension for "habitual intoxication and providing professional services while under the influence of alcohol." Another was suspended for leaving an anesthetized patient unattended and then, apparently, providing misleading testimony in an investigation of the incident.

My doctor wasn't lucky enough to receive a suspension. In fact, in Dr. Rothstein's case "the Board will not consider any reapplication for 5 years." In other words, for using unconventional treatments, he was put in the same group as a murderer. But a doctor who treated her patients while intoxicated received a suspension. When her suspension is lifted, she'll continue to practice while under probation.

It's beyond belief! You can be drunk while treating patients and receive a lighter punishment than if you effectively treat patients by using methods that are outside of the narrow mainstream definition of healthcare.

You call THAT medicine?

In the official ruling, Dr. Rothstein's license was revoked for practicing "substandard medicine." I personally have been a victim of his "substandard" treatments for almost 3 years now—and have been willing to pay out-of-pocket to subject myself to them.

My back and neck seized up so badly one weekend that I literally cried just trying to sit down on my bed. I had to cancel a speaking engagement and could barely move. My husband carefully got me into the car and took me to Dr. Rothstein's office, where this "quack" realized that my diaphragm was in spasm and released it. After 48 hours of being nearly immobile, my pain completely disappeared in less than 30 minutes. It was truly astonishing.

Dr. Rothstein isn't one of those doctors who knows what's wrong with you before you come in or has a prescription pad at the ready so he can send you on your way 10 minutes later and feel he's done his job. He takes an extraordinary amount of time to work with patients and listen to them—a skill few doctors exhibit these days.

Unfortunately, the belief that taking 15 extra minutes and releasing a diaphragm in spasm is actually better treatment than a handful of muscle relaxers and a week of lying in bed makes you dangerous in the state of Maryland—a state where if you go around healing people rather than medicating them you're punished as if you were a convicted murderer.

Legal eagles

It's important to note again that Dr. Rothstein has had no complaints from patients lodged against him. And I'm not surprised. Personally I am devastated that I can't go to his office for treatment anymore. Professionally, I am outraged that this skilled healer is being targeted by an overzealous medical establishment that is clearly threatened by any ideas outside of its very small box.

The truth is that Dr. Rothstein will likely go on and prosper regardless of how this chapter ends. He is a wonderfully talented man with a strong support network and an equally strong constitution. So the real victims of the Maryland Board of Physicians are the very patients they claim they are trying to protect—the ones who will no longer be able to get real, honest, caring medical treatment from a man they trust who knows that patients aren't just insurance ID numbers that appear in 15 minute increments.

...and another thing

There used to be a large Wonder Bread bakery in South Miami, and although their product was the blandest food known to man, the aroma in that neighborhood always had the sweet pungency that apparently turns automobile drivers into crazy people.

I'm not sure what the rate of accidents was in South Miami during the 60s and 70s, but it may have been much higher than the rest of the city. According to research from the RAC Foundation for Motoring (a UK advocacy group for safe driving), the aroma of freshly baked bread can prompt a driver to turn surly and drive at higher speeds. The aroma of fast food has the same effect.

So when you see cars pulling out of MacDonald's or Burger King drive-thrus, it might be wise to give them a wide berth.

The results of this study brought to mind the e-Alert "Every Size Fits All" (6/22/05) in which I told you about the campaign known as HAES, or "health at every size." The HAES program encourages plus-sized folks to accept and respect their body type while shifting their dietary focus from weight loss to pursuing good health. But to do that, you have to recognize the triggers that can set off eating binges.

Conrad King, a psychologist and one of the authors of the RAC study, told Food Navigator-USA that the sense of smell "circumnavigates the logical part of the brain" and plays directly on emotions. So put a cardboard container of French fries in the car, and your reaction might turn emotional, bypassing good dietary logic. Against your better judgment you might hear yourself say, "Pass the fries, please. NOW!"

Or you could have a mint instead of fries. The RAC study also found that certain aromas—such as peppermint, coffee, lemon and cinnamon—improved drivers' temperaments and sharpened concentration. Maybe those aromas could also help us avoid losing our heads and impulsively chowing down when we know we really shouldn't.

To Your Good Health,

Jenny Thompson
Health Sciences Institute

Sources:

- "Smell of Fresh Bread and Fast Food Influences Behaviour" Lindsey Partos, Food Navigator-USA, 6/10/05, foodnavigator-usa.com

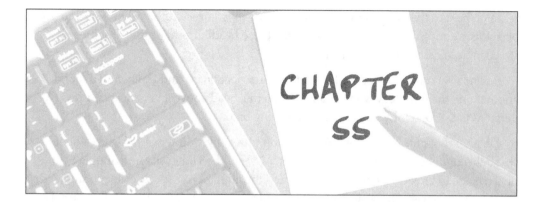

Blind man's bluff: The dark mysteries of erectile dysfunction

First ran 7/20/2005

Life is full of surprises. For instance, if you're a man who uses one of the popular medications that address erectile dysfunction (ED), you and Bob Dole could be in for a very unpleasant surprise. But before we examine the dark mysteries of ED drugs, let's see what happens when a researcher researches research.

The headliner

Long-time e-Alert readers may have noticed that one of my pet peeves is the wild inaccuracy often found in news headlines. When a headline writer states that vitamin E, for instance, is "proven" to have no beneficial effects on heart health, and then the research behind the news item turns out to be deeply flawed…that's when I see red. At best, this is simply lazy and sloppy. At worst, these headlines may mislead some consumers into making poor health choices.

So I'm always on the lookout for off-the-mark headlines. And I thought I'd found another one the other day when I came across this head above an Associated Press (AP) item: "What's 'good for you' often ends up being bad."

Uh oh, I thought. Here we go. But instead I found a very interesting article about research, conducted by John P. A. Ioannidis, M.D., of the University of Ioannina School of Medicine in Greece. Dr. Ioannidis searched through more than a decade of studies published in Lancet, The New England Journal of Medicine (NEJM), and the Journal of the American Medical Association (JAMA; where, coincidentally, Dr. Ioannidis' study was published earlier this month).

Dr. Ioannidis found nearly 50 original clinical research studies that had repeated follow up studies published between 1990 and 2003. Forty-five of the original studies concluded that the treatment being researched was effective. But in the follow-ups, 16 percent concluded that the treatments were ineffective, while another 16 percent concluded that the effects of treatment were stronger than the original studies found them to be.

In the AP article the editors of NEJM noted how important it is to recognize that, "A single study is not the final word."—an outlook I've frequently expressed in the e-Alert.

But my favorite quote in the article comes from Catherine DeAngelis; the editor of JAMA, who told the AP that matters get even more complicated when the media produces "misleading or exaggerated headlines." With you all the way on that one, Dr. D!

Case in point

To illustrate Dr. Ioannidis' point about needing more than just one study to uncover the full range of pros and cons of a treatment, we only need to look at a drug that's received more than 100 clinical trials. That's right—it's the wildly popular erectile dysfunction drug that has achieved cultural icon status in less than a decade: Viagra.

According to a Washington Post article, NONE of those 100+ trials picked up on a rare but severe side effect of the drug: Men who have diabetes, hypertension or high cholesterol may experience sudden partial blindness. This past spring the Journal of Neuro-Ophthalmology carried a report that examined seven men, aged 50 to 70, who developed this side effect—known as nonarteritic anterior ischemic optic neuropathy

(NAION)—within 36 hours of taking Viagra. In some cases, vision wasn't completely restored.

In addition, the Post reports that the FDA has received more than 35 complaints from Viagra users who suffered sudden and permanent loss of sight in one eye. CBS News claims that number may be much higher: perhaps more than 100 cases.

As a result of this surprising development the FDA has "approved updated labeling" for Viagra and other ED drugs. This note appeared in last week's FDA News Digest: "FDA urges patients taking these drugs who experience sudden vision loss or decreased vision in one or both eyes to stop taking the drug and contact a medical professional right away."

It's priceless: If everything suddenly goes dark or blurry or blue, just read (or attempt to read) the information sheet that came with the medication; printed in microscopic typeface, of course. And then try to find the phone to call your doctor.

It's hard to say what treatment a doctor might suggest for this unique condition, but you can bet he probably won't be aware that an FDA safety officer informed her superiors of the blindness danger more than a YEAR before the Journal of Neuro-Ophthalmology study was published (according to the Post).

In the bureaucratic mind, information isn't power, regulation is power. FDA officials can't just issue a well-publicized statement when they detect an obvious danger. They have to sit on the information while the wheels of bureaucracy slowly grind out a requirement for a warning on the drug's information sheet.

So if you know any men who use Viagra, Levitra or Cialis, give them the news that will eventually be mentioned somewhere on drug information sheets: When these medications are taken by those with diabetes, hypertension or high cholesterol, there's a chance that everything might go dim. Permanently.

...and another thing

When you're puzzling over menu options, here's one more reason to order that curry dish...

Curcumin is a yellow pigment in the root of turmeric, an herb in the ginger family. Curry gets its distinct color and flavor from curcumin, which was used by Indian

Ayurvedic healers for thousands of years to treat a variety of ailments, including indigestion, jaundice, arthritis, and urinary tract disorders.

A recent issue of the journal Cancer reports on a study from the University of Texas where researchers treated melanoma cell lines with curcumin, which caused cell function to decrease. Various concentrations of curcumin also prompted tumor cell apoptosis (self destruction of cancer cells) by suppressing proteins that prevent apoptosis.

This isn't the first time we've seen beneficial effects from curcumin. In previous e-Alerts I've told you how this pigment may also inhibit angiogenesis; the process by which cancer cells thrive by creating tiny blood vessels.

And curcumin may also help prevent dementia. In recent years, studies have shown that curcumin's antioxidant and anti-inflammatory properties may be powerful enough to break up the amyloid plaques in the brain that contribute to Alzheimer's disease. The rate of Alzheimer's in India (where turmeric is widely consumed) is among the lowest in the world.

To Your Good Health,

Jenny Thompson
Health Sciences Institute

Sources:

- "What's 'Good For You' Often Ends Up Being Bad" The Associated Press, 7/12/05, msnbc.com
- "Contradicted and Initially Stronger Effects in Highly Cited Clinical Research" Journal of the American Medical Association, Vol. 294, No. 2, 7/13/05, jama.ama-assn.org
- "FDA Was Told of Viagra-Blindness Link Months Ago" Marc Kaufman, Washington Post, 7/1/05, washingtonpost.com
- "Reports of Eye Problems Prompt Label Change for Impotence Drugs" FDA News Digest, 7/11/05, list.nih.gov
- "Turmeric Slows Melanoma Growth in Lab Study" NutraIngredients.com, 7/11/05, nutraingredients.com

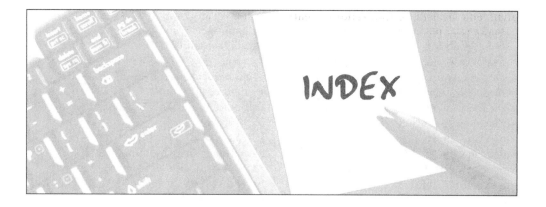

INDEX

Engaging Commentary, Unique Perspectives, and the Health News You Will Not Hear About Anywhere Else

Now you can receive the Health Sciences Institute's exclusive e-Alerts, sent directly from the desk of Jenny Thompson to your in-box...ABSOLUTELY FREE! If you enjoyed this book and would like to read more of the engaging commentary and unique perspectives of Jenny Thompson you saw here you can now sign up for the e-Alert, normally sent only to HSI members, for free.

Each day, we receive hundreds of e-mails from readers letting us know we are on the right track. They tell us they don't get this kind of insightful information anywhere else. Here are just a few examples of what our readers have said to us lately:

- *Boris S. wrote, "Thank you again for your updates and alerts. You have been consistent and perfect," following our story on the food industry's attempt to introduce natural bacteria killers.*

- *Ruth W. wrote to say, "What a wonderful report on NIH ignoring the true cause(s) of disease," after reading our alert about NIH's decision to lower standards for high cholesterol, in turn recommending drugs for millions more Americans.*

- *And Dr. Fritz writes: "Your e-mails, just as your newsletter, are most important for me. Thank you for what you are doing for your members."*

Sign up for FREE today!

Signing up is incredibly simple. Just visit www.hsibaltimore.com and let us know where you'd like your copy of the e-Alert sent. Shortly after you will receive a welcome e-mail from Jenny and then your e-Alerts will start coming directly to your in box.

We share your concerns over privacy. HSI will never sell your e-mail address. And, of course, you can unsubscribe at any time.